Infant Safe Sleep

T0171893

Rachel Y. Moon
Editor

Infant Safe Sleep

A Pocket Guide for Clinicians

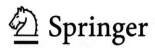 Springer

Editor
Rachel Y. Moon
University of Virginia
Charlottesville, VA
USA

ISBN 978-3-030-47541-3   ISBN 978-3-030-47542-0   (eBook)
https://doi.org/10.1007/978-3-030-47542-0

This Springer imprint is published by the registered company Springer Nature Switzerland AG
The registered company address is: Gewerbestrasse 11, 6330 Cham, Switzerland

Dedication
To Steve, Sarah, and Elizabeth
For always and forever
With love and gratitude

Preface

The death of a healthy baby – there is not much worse than that. Every year in the USA, nearly 3600 babies die suddenly and unexpectedly. That is 3600 babies too many. Each of these babies has a name. For their parents, it is the nightmare that never ends. For every person who has ever touched that baby, physically or figuratively – whether it be a relative, child care provider, friend, nurse, physician, or other person – it is a tragedy that stays with them for a very, very long time.

I have spent most of my professional life studying the risk factors that are associated with these sudden and unexpected deaths, talking with parents and health care professionals to better understand why people may or may not follow safe sleep recommendations, and testing specific interventions to try to change parent practice.

In this book, I have tried to compile the practical, evidence-based information that clinicians need to most effectively talk with parents about safe sleep. If you don't understand why these babies die (or our best knowledge about why these babies die), then the safe sleep guidelines will not make much sense. Thus, there is a chapter about pathophysiology of these deaths. If you don't understand how people make decisions, then you may have more difficulty selling the safe sleep message. Thus, there is a chapter about decision-making. If you don't know what parents' concerns are – or what others around them are recommending – you will not be able to address those concerns. If you don't address the concerns, you have very little chance of convincing them to change what they're doing. Thus, there is a chapter for each of the sleep environment components. There are also chapters that discuss special situations (premature babies, babies with gastro-esophageal reflux, etc.) and what to do if one of your families does lose a baby. It is my hope that this book helps you navigate all of these discussions.

I would like to thank my colleagues who work in this line of research. There are not many of us who work in the field of SIDS and SUID, and we are a fairly close-knit group. Many of these colleagues – Sam Hanke, Rosemary Horne, Trina Salm Ward, Bryanne Colvin, Eve Colson, Fern Hauck, Ann Kellams, Rebecca Carlin, Jeffrey Colvin, Michael Goodstein, and Rick Goldstein – have taken the time and energy to write chapters for this book, and they get an extra-special thank you. You cannot work in this field without becoming passionate about it, and these colleagues are all that. It is often hard to find good work friends – but in this field, I have been fortunate to have many. We work hard together, but also have enjoyed many a meal (and a few glasses of wine!) together. I am proud and humbled to call them all my colleagues – and my friends.

I want to end by thanking the families who have lost babies. You have become members of this club that nobody wants to be a member of. You come to conferences to ask questions and learn more, you make sure that your younger children know about their older brother or sister, and you bravely share your stories so that other parents never have to go through this. Your stories and your dedication to this cause inspire me every single day. You are my heroes.

Charlottesville, VA, USA   Rachel Y. Moon

Editor's Note About Nomenclature

For multiple reasons, over the past 15–20 years, there has been a shift in diagnostic terminology for babies who have died suddenly and unexpectedly, usually in a sleep setting. The predominant diagnosis used for cause of death determination has traditionally been sudden infant death syndrome (SIDS). In recent years, this term has been largely replaced in the medical literature with sudden unexpected infant death (SUID) or sudden unexpected death in infancy (SUDI). SUID is the term that is used when an infant dies suddenly and unexpectedly, and implies the preliminary diagnosis before the death investigation, including autopsy, scene investigation, and review of clinical history, is performed. Following the investigation, some of the deaths will be determined to have a natural cause, e.g., infection or cardiac disease. The other deaths will be attributed to SIDS (~50%), accidental suffocation and strangulation in bed (ASSB) (~25%), and ill-defined/unknown/undetermined cause of death (~25%). Because of inconsistencies in the evidence required for these different categories, they are grouped together and referred to (also) as SUID, which in this case means sudden unexplained infant death, since they have gone through complete autopsies and death scene investigations without revealing an explanation sufficient to determine cause. Thus, when one reads any published work on this topic, it is important to first determine what acronyms are being used and how they are defined.

These changes in the use of diagnostic categories, referred to as "diagnostic shift," have led to a simultaneous decrease in the SIDS rate and increases in rates of ASSB and ill-defined/unknown/undetermined. Because the risk factors, the autopsy findings, and the death scene investigations for these 3 diagnoses are very similar, and because safe sleep guidelines reduce the risk of all 3 causes of death, public health campaigns have targeted all of these deaths. These deaths, because they mostly occur in a sleep environment or during sleep, are also referred to as *sleep-related infant deaths*. You will see all of these terms in this book.

Research from before 2000 largely refers to SIDS. However, it should be understood by the reader that at least a proportion of these deaths would likely now be attributed to ASSB or ill-defined/unknown/undetermined. Research published after 2000 increasingly uses the terms SUID, SUDI, or sleep-related infant deaths. The lack of consistency in how these deaths are certified and coded (with ICD-10 codes) has complicated research and prevention efforts – after all, if there is no consistency in what these deaths are called, it is difficult to conduct research and create interventions, as you do not know if these efforts are resulting in improvements.

There are continuing efforts to standardize the nomenclature. The 3rd International Congress on Sudden Infant and Child Death, comprised of pediatricians, pediatric pathologists, forensic pathologists, family physicians, epidemiologists, statisticians, researchers, and parents representatives, was convened in November 2019 to make recommendations to the World Health Organization for revisions in ICD coding that would ideally standardize nomenclature in the ICD-11. There was consensus to propose a title change from "SIDS" to "Unexplained Sudden Infant Death in Infancy or SIDS," and explicit guidance for death certifiers regarding use of the alternative categories of "accidental asphyxia" and "undetermined." At the time of publication of this book, decision by the World Health Organization is pending.

Contents

Contributors

Rebecca Carlin, MD Columbia University, New York, NY, USA

Eve R. Colson, MD, MHPE Washington University in St. Louis School of Medicine, St. Louis, MO, USA

Bryanne N. Colvin, MD Washington University in St. Louis School of Medicine, St. Louis, MO, USA

Jeffrey D. Colvin, MD, JD Pediatrics, Children's Mercy Kansas City, Kansas City, MO, USA

Richard D. Goldstein, MD Robert's Program on Sudden Unexpected Death in Pediatrics, Division of General Pediatrics, Department of Pediatrics, Boston Children's Hospital and Harvard Medical School, Boston, MA, USA

Michael Goodstein, MD, FAAP Pediatrics, WellSpan York Hospital, York, PA, USA

Samuel Hanke, MD, MS Heart Institute, Cincinnati Children's Hospital Medical Center, Cincinnati, OH, USA

Fern R. Hauck, MD, MS Department of Family Medicine, University of Virginia, Charlottesville, VA, USA

Rosemary S. C. Horne, BSc, MSc, PhD, BLitt, DSc Department of Paediatrics, Monash University, Melbourne, VIC, Australia

Ann Kellams, MD University of Virginia, Department of Pediatrics, Charlottesville, VA, USA

Rachel Y. Moon, MD Department of Pediatrics, University of Virginia School of Medicine, Charlottesville, VA, USA

Trina C. Salm Ward, PhD, MSW Department of Social Work, Helen Bader School of Social Welfare, University of Wisconsin-Milwaukee, Milwaukee, WI, USA

Chapter 1
Why This Book
Is Important

Samuel Hanke

Safe Sleep Chose Me

The night my son died started out as an average evening in late April. My wife, Maura, and I were 3 weeks into our new roles as mom and dad, navigating the challenges that come with parenting an infant. We were learning and loving every moment of those first 21 days – keeping track of his feedings and trying to master the ins and outs of diapering, burping, and swaddling. We snapped photos of his first smile, his first bath, and the first time he met Gramps.

From the moment he was born on April 6, 2010, he was an absolute joy and light of our lives. He was healthy and beautiful – absolutely perfect. We named him Charlie Paul (Fig. 1.1).

Eager to do our best, we quickly figured out how our son liked to be held after feedings. We prayed over him and poured all of our energy into making sure our baby boy had enough – enough milk, enough love, enough comfort, and enough safety. As a pediatrician and Maura a kindergarten teacher, we thought we had a leg up.

S. Hanke (✉)
Heart Institute, Cincinnati Children's Hospital Medical Center, Cincinnati, OH, USA
e-mail: Samuel.hanke@cchmc.org

© Springer Nature Switzerland AG 2020
R. Y. Moon (ed.), *Infant Safe Sleep*,
https://doi.org/10.1007/978-3-030-47542-0_1

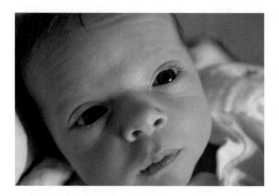

FIGURE 1.1 Charlie Paul Hanke at 2 weeks old

Charlie, like most newborns, needed help getting the sleep thing down. Nightly bouts of crying came at the expense of sleep for his mom and dad.

On that particular evening in April, Maura, who exclusively breastfed Charlie, was exhausted from what felt like the hourly ritual of feeding, burping, changing, repeat. So, I tagged in on dad duty.

I scooped a fussy Charlie up from his bare crib and sat down on the couch to soothe him back to sleep – SportsCenter™ serving as the quiet soundtrack on the TV. Imagine the picture of sleep-deprived father and son. It wasn't unusual; we often see this photo on social media – baby asleep on dad's chest, dad accidentally dozes off to sleep too. That was me.

But when I woke up – Charlie didn't.

In that one moment, Charlie's life ended and the entire trajectory of mine changed. I went from a sleep-deprived father watching ESPN™ with my son to a grieving one. That one minute in time – fueled by exhaustion and a desire to do what was best for my baby – changed every notion I had about how life was supposed to play out.

A decade has passed, and Maura and I continue to feel the pain from the impact of that night.

In the time since Charlie's death, we have spent countless hours reflecting on the questions. What didn't we know?

What could we tell others to do differently? And how can we help new parents to make sure they don't suffer the same tragic loss?

We Are Not Alone

Approximately 3600 babies die every year in the United States due to sleep-related infant death – an average of one baby's death every 2 hours. These babies leave behind devastated families, like mine, spanning every state, every race, and every socioeconomic group.

In fact, sleep-related infant death kills more under-18-year-old American children than opioids, gun violence, car accidents, or suicides (Fig. 1.2). But where is the story?

One only needs to turn on the news to see the public outcry demanding action against the reprehensible eruption of

U.S. under-18 deaths by cause, 2017

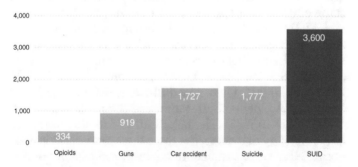

FIGURE 1.2 Selected US under-18 deaths, by ICD-10 cause of death, in 2017 (the most recent year available). Centers for Disease Control and Prevention, National Center for Health Statistics. Multiple Cause of Death 1999–2017 on CDC WONDER Online Database, released December, 2018. (Data are from the Multiple Cause of Death Files, 1999–2017, as compiled from data provided by the 57 vital statistics jurisdictions through the Vital Statistics Cooperative Program. Accessed at http://wonder.cdc.gov/mcd-icd10.html. Reproduced with permission from Bill Rapp)

gun violence. The American people and politicians focus a great deal of attention on gun safety – and should. Outrage is appropriate when children die. We should be screaming from the rooftops for change.

Sadly, there is no public outcry for the nearly 4000 babies who are dying year in and year out. Why is this?

SIDS, SUID, ASSB: The Alphabet Soup of Sleep-Related Deaths

How can we move the needle when the needle keeps changing? As providers, the first problem we need to fix is that our patients may not understand what we are asking them to prevent.

We promote safe sleep practices to combat SUID (Sudden Unexpected Infant Death), which is defined as the death of an infant (i.e., someone who is younger than 365 days of age) that occurs suddenly and unexpectedly and for which the cause of death is not immediately obvious prior to investigation. SUID is used as the term before the autopsy and death scene investigation are completed, after which three diagnoses recognized in ICD-10 coding are generally used as cause of death: Sudden Infant Death Syndrome (SIDS; ICD-10 R95), Unknown/Undetermined/Ill-Defined Causes (ICD-10 R99), and Accidental Suffocation and Strangulation in Bed (ASSB; ICD-10 W75) (Fig. 1.3). SUID is also often used as a broad category that comprises these three more specific diagnoses. Because the vast majority of these deaths occur during sleep or in a sleep environment, they are also referred to as sleep-related infant deaths.

Why is this distinction important? Because many believe that Sudden Infant Death Syndrome (SIDS) is a problem that was solved and that no longer exists. SIDS, which is defined as the unexpected death of an infant under 1 year of age, for which no cause of death could be determined after a thorough investigation, including death scene, autopsy, and medical history, is the cause of death that was traditionally given

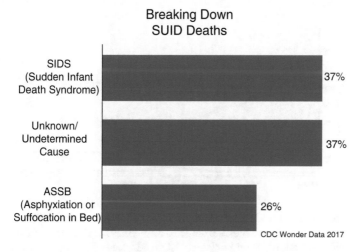

FIGURE 1.3 SUID sleep-related infant deaths by category in 2017. (Data from the Centers for Disease Control and Prevention. CDC Wonder. http://wonder.cdc.gov/)

to most infants who died suddenly and unexpectedly. However, in recent years, for a number of reasons, including improved standardization of death scene investigations and a growing reluctance among some death certifiers to use "SIDS" as a cause of death, many deaths that would have been coded as SIDS 20 years ago are being coded differently today.

Thus, the decline in SIDS rates does not reflect the reality. When we look at the overall picture (Fig. 1.4), although SIDS rates have dropped, the rates of other causes of SUID have risen, such that the overall SUID rate has remained stagnant since the beginning of the century.

We also need to realize that because SIDS is defined as a death for which no reason can be found, many parents believe that SIDS occurs randomly or is "God's will" and thus will reason that there is no point in following safe sleep recommendations [1]. Parents may feel powerless against something like this occurring. When these infants do die in their sleep, it is often handled as a quiet, personal, and private

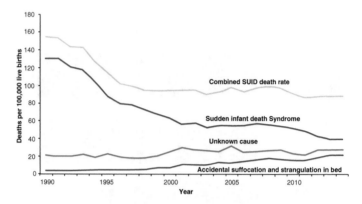

FIGURE 1.4 Trends in Sudden Unexpected Infant Death (SUID) rates in the United States from 1990 through 2017. (Data from CDC/NCHS, National Vital Statistics System, Mortality Files. https://www.cdc.gov/sids/data.htm. Courtesy of CDC/NCHS)

suffering. However, given that every year in the United States, 3600 otherwise healthy infants go to bed and do not wake up ever again, it is a public health crisis.

We know that these deaths, whether they are called SIDS or something else, most often occur in the presence of known risk factors (see Fig. 1.5). (Take my case, for example. While Charlie's cause of death was SIDS, known risk factors were present.) We also know that elimination of these risk factors vastly reduces a baby's SUID risk.

We as providers must share this information with parents, so that they will feel empowered, not powerless against SUID.

Room for Improvement

Reassuringly, our patients continue to listen to our advice. Numerous studies have demonstrated that despite the increasing influences of other voices in our society, provider recommendation is the primary influencer of sleep position and location [3]. Unfortunately, the majority of our patients

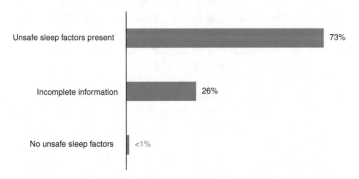

FIGURE 1.5 Fewer than 1% of SUID deaths occur when the baby is supine, on a flat sleep surface in a crib or bassinet, with no unsafe sleep factors. (Adapted from Ref. [2])

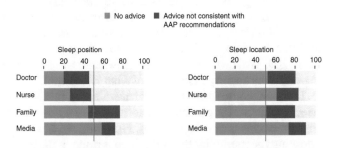

FIGURE 1.6 On the topics of sleep position and sleep location, many parents continue to receive inappropriate advice or lack of advice [5]. (Reproduced with permission from Bill Rapp)

are not hearing the evidence-based American Academy of Pediatrics' recommendations from us (Fig. 1.6) [4]. We cannot impact parents if we don't talk about it. Additionally, if we don't talk about it, parents may infer that the recommendations are not important.

However, this is an easily modifiable practice. If providers make time for these important conversations about safe sleep, we can most likely change outcomes. Health-care providers have an essential role in making sure families are intimately aware of the risks they are taking when it comes to infant sleep and preventing SUID.

It is my belief that parents don't know, or probably more accurately, don't understand the risks they are taking, and therefore lack motivation and follow-through. Health-care providers, in partnership with families and communities, have the knowledge and the power to change things. For instance, coaching parents to understand that they should not expect a newborn to sleep more than 2–3 hours at a stretch can help them set reasonable expectations when making a late-night feeding plan to combat exhaustion.

Unfortunately, societal pressures suggest a sleeping infant is the gold standard for successful baby parenting. New parents are asked from nearly day one, "is your baby sleeping through the night?" Of course, we know that no neonate should sleep all night long, because infants need to eat every few hours. Even more important for new parents to understand is that babies who sleep flat on their backs wake more frequently – and that this improved arousability puts them at a lower risk for SUID. We have to share this knowledge to reset parental expectations and understanding of what is "normal."

I am writing to you as a pediatrician and a father to show people that SUID can happen to anyone. I know firsthand that practicing safe sleep is hard. However, we have to start adopting the mentality that safe sleep is nonnegotiable. I cannot emphasize enough that practicing safe sleep for every sleep is as important as buckling your child in a car seat for every drive.

Practical Questions and Advice

We know that, when practiced, the safe sleep guidelines save lives.

But solving the issue of sleep-related infant death is more than just preaching these guidelines. It is about making sure the caregivers in our communities follow them, even when they feel impossibly hard.

In order to do that, providers need to share real solutions to help them be successful. How are we going to help a single, working mother suffering from exhaustion to consistently practice safe sleep?

We may have the best intentions for our babies, but it takes one time, one judgment call in a moment of fatigue to pull a baby into the parental bed, or in my case, lie down on the couch, and put our infants at risk.

As health-care providers, we need to talk about the challenges and the exhaustion new parents face and what we can do to combat them. When we disseminate safe sleep information with real practical tips, we can quite literally save a life.

Think about examples of specific questions to ask new parents.

Do you have support when it comes to breastfeeding your baby?

Do you have a crib? When do you use it?

What are others in your life telling you about where and how the baby should sleep?

Do you have someone who can take care of the baby when you need to sleep?

Once you understand where the struggle to practice safe sleep resides, you can begin to form a narrative for how to support each family. Effective teaching starts with empathy, so hearing the problems allows you to make a plan with parents to overcome them.

Real Stories, Real Families

In addition to pointed questions and practical tips, we also need to show families why it is important, by sharing real stories from those in our community who have been impacted by sleep-related deaths.

That's why I'm writing this chapter. The "why" we need to practice safe sleep is deeply personal to me. My why is my son, Charlie.

Sadly, there are thousands of families just like mine who have suffered infant loss. Recognize and share stories of real families to help families connect with this crisis.

Did you know that Shaun Alexander, Hall of Fame NFL superstar, lost a child to SUID? He and his wife have ten beautiful children [6]. Their ninth child, a precious girl named Torah, was placed for a nap the way they slept all of their children – on an adult bed on her stomach. Since all of their other babies had been fine sleeping this way, they didn't think anything of it, until tragically she never woke up.

Since losing Torah, the Alexanders have welcomed their tenth child and are vigilant about safe sleep. They are firm believers that safe sleep could have saved Torah's life.

For too many parents, SUID is something that happens to other families. The average American is unaware that ten babies in the United States die every single day. Worse, many parents and grandparents don't understand that the common denominator of these deaths is a lack of adherence to safe sleep practices.

As clinicians we must recognize that saving these infants does not require a diagnosis but rather a communication strategy.

It Starts with a List of Recommendations

The 2016 AAP Recommendations are a vital, evidence-based foundation for safe sleep standards [7]. But these detailed recommendations are far removed from the singular vital behavior promoted by the profoundly effective *Back to Sleep* campaign in the mid-1990s. It is up to health-care providers to digest, understand, and distill the information needed most by parents and caregivers in a way that is simple, direct, and achievable.

Instead of recommending parents practice safe sleep, we should insist upon it. And with that insistence, normalize infant sleep needs, and provide suggestions to removing barriers that make safe sleep difficult.

Parents will ultimately make choices for their child based on their own set of beliefs. However, if directives are clear and success is celebrated, we have a real shot at connecting with parents even when they are their most vulnerable. The interaction parents have with you during their visit just might replay in their minds when they are tired and desperate for sleep. When we as providers are strong in our convictions, parents can be strong when exhaustion sets in and choices are made.

If you need a place to start, consider using a tool like the book, *Sleep Baby Safe and Snug* (Fig. 1.7). When my wife and I started Charlie's Kids Foundation in 2011, we wanted to

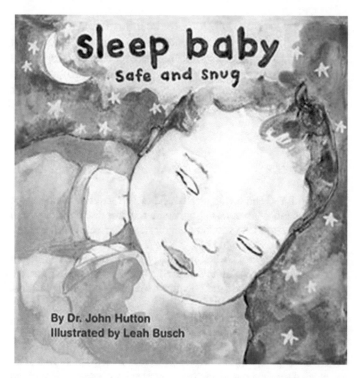

FIGURE 1.7 Front cover of the Charlie's Kids Foundation book, Sleep Baby Safe and Snug, that is used to teach parents and caregivers about infant safe sleep. Charlie's Kids Foundation, 2019

provide resources for new parents about infant safe sleep so that other families would not have to suffer through a similar loss.

We created *Sleep Baby Safe and Snug* to share the AAP safe sleep recommendations in a simple and different form, one that we know is helping providers to open the conversation about safe sleep in a non-threatening way. Since then, we have distributed over 3.5 million books across the country via hospitals, pediatricians, community advocacy groups, and state health departments.

Through this small but important book, we know Charlie is making a big difference and saving lives [8–10]. But *ALL* of us can too.

My hope is that you will share the information in this book and our story with the parents and caregivers whom you encounter. Encourage them to practice safe sleep. And when it feels especially hard and they feel the exhaustion that often comes with being a new parent, encourage them ask their partners/families/friends for help, remember Charlie, and keep their baby safe.

References

1. Moon RY, Oden RP, Joyner BL, Ajao TI. Qualitative analysis of beliefs and perceptions about sudden infant death syndrome in African-American mothers: implications for safe sleep recommendations. J Pediatr. 2010;157(1):92–7.e2.
2. Shapiro-Mendoza CK, Camperlengo L, Ludvigsen R, Cottengim C, Anderson RN, Andrew T, et al. Classification system for the sudden unexpected infant death case registry and its application. Pediatrics. 2014;134(1):e210–e9.
3. Vernacchio L, Corwin MJ, Lesko SM, Vezina RM, Hunt CE, Hoffman HJ, et al. Sleep position of low birth weight infants. Pediatrics. 2003;111(3):633–40.
4. Hirai AH, Kortsmit K, Kaplan L, Reiney E, Warner L, Parks SE, et al. Prevalence and factors associated with safe infant sleep practices. Pediatrics. 2019;144:e20191286.

5. Eisenberg SR, Bair-Merritt MH, Colson ER, Heeren TC, Geller NL, Corwin MJ. Maternal report of advice received for infant care. Pediatrics. 2015;136(2):e315–e22.

6. Cradle Cincinnati. The Alexander family on the loss of their infant and safe sleep. YouTube. 2018. youtu.be/ch9rjZy4Kww.

7. Moon RY, Syndrome TFoSID. SIDS and other sleep-related infant deaths: evidence base for 2016 updated recommendations for a safe infant sleeping environment. Pediatrics. 2016;138(5):e20162940.

8. Hutton JS, Gupta R, Gruber R, Berndsen J, DeWitt T, Ollberding NJ, et al. Randomized trial of a children's book versus brochures for safe sleep knowledge and adherence in a high-risk population. Acad Pediatr. 2017;17(8):879–86.

9. Heitmann R, Nilles EK, Jeans A, Moreland J, Clarke C, McDonald MF, et al. Improving safe sleep modeling in the hospital through policy implementation. Matern Child Health J. 2017;21(11):1995–2000.

10. Walcott R, Ward TS, Ingels J, Llewellyn N, Miller T, Corso P. A statewide hospital-based safe infant sleep initiative: measurement of parental knowledge and behavior. J Community Health. 2018;43(3):534–42.

Chapter 2
How Pathophysiology Explains Risk and Protective Factors

Rosemary S. C. Horne

Introduction

Sudden infant death syndrome (SIDS) is currently defined as "the sudden unexpected death of an infant <1 year of age, with onset of the fatal episode apparently occurring during sleep, that remains unexplained after a thorough investigation, including performance of a complete autopsy and review of the circumstances of death and the clinical history" [1]. Recently, the terms sudden unexpected infant death (SUID) and sudden unexpected death in infancy (SUDI) have largely replaced SIDS in the medical literature. These terms refer to the unexpected death of an infant, usually occurring during sleep, in which a cause of death is not immediately obvious. SUID and SUDI are essentially research classifications (i.e., are not in the ICD-10 classification system and thus not generally used for cause of death certification). The terms refer to a broad category of sudden and unexpected deaths, which include SIDS, infections or anatomical or developmental abnormalities not recognized before death,

R. S. C. Horne (✉)
Department of Paediatrics, Monash University, Melbourne, VIC, Australia
e-mail: rosemary.horne@monash.edu

© Springer Nature Switzerland AG 2020
R. Y. Moon (ed.), *Infant Safe Sleep*,
https://doi.org/10.1007/978-3-030-47542-0_2

accidental suffocation or strangulation in bed, unknown/ undetermined/ill-defined causes of death, and sudden unexpected deaths that are revealed by investigations to have been the result of non-accidental injuries.

There has been considerable research into the underlying mechanisms that may underpin known risk factors. SIDS is believed to be multifactorial in origin. The triple risk hypothesis has been proposed to explain this [2]. The model proposes that when a vulnerable infant, such as one born preterm or exposed to maternal smoking, is at a critical but unstable developmental period in homeostatic control (the highest risk period is 2–4 months, with 90% of deaths occurring before 6 months) and is exposed to an exogenous stressor, such as being placed prone for sleep, then death may occur (Fig. 2.1). The model proposes that infants will die only if all three factors are present and that the vulnerability lies dormant until the infant enters the critical developmental period and is exposed to an exogenous stressor. SIDS occurs during sleep, and the peak incidence is between 2 and 4 months of age, when sleep patterns and cardiorespiratory control are rapidly maturing. *The final pathway to SIDS is widely believed to involve some combination of immature cardiorespiratory control and a failure of arousal from sleep.*

Arousal from sleep is a vital protective response [3]. When we go to sleep, heart rate and blood pressure fall, breathing slows, and responses to hypoxic and hypercapnic stimuli are reduced. Simply by arousing from sleep, heart rate, blood pressure, and breathing are increased. Importantly, behavioral responses, such as turning the head to remove bedding or to uncover the nose and mouth if sleeping prone, can be initiated during arousal from sleep. Support for the failure of the cardiorespiratory/arousal hypothesis comes from numerous physiological studies showing that the major risk factors for SIDS (prone sleeping, maternal smoking, prematurity, head covering) both impair arousal from sleep and have significant adverse effects on blood pressure and heart rate and their control. Conversely, protective factors (breastfeeding, immunization, and use of a pacifier) are associated with improved cardiorespiratory control and arousability [4].

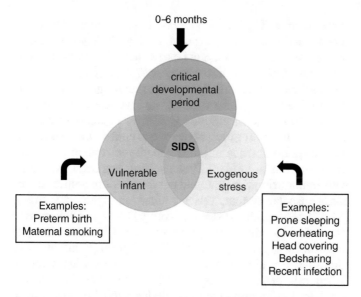

FIGURE 2.1 Triple risk model for SIDS illustrating the three overlapping factors: (1) a vulnerable infant, (2) a critical developmental period, and (3) an exogenous stress. (Adapted from Ref. [2]). This model proposes that when a vulnerable infant, for example, one born preterm or exposed to maternal smoking, is at a critical but unstable developmental period in homeostatic control and is exposed to an exogenous stressor, such as being placed prone to sleep, overheated, having their head covered, are in a bed-sharing situation, or have recently had an infection, then death may occur

Why Are Infants Vulnerable to Cardiorespiratory Challenges?

A number of significant developmental factors may make an infant more vulnerable to a cardiorespiratory challenge during the critical developmental period from birth to 6 months of age – and particularly between 2 and 4 months – when the risk of SIDS is highest.

Autonomic control increases with gestational age in the fetus during pregnancy [5, 6]. Both parasympathetic and sympathetic activities increase during gestation, but not in the same manner. The largest increase in parasympathetic activity occurs during the last trimester, while the largest increase in sympathetic activity occurs early on, with smaller changes occurring during the last trimester [7]. After birth at term, heart rate increases initially over the first month of life before declining gradually, as a result of an increase in parasympathetic dominance of autonomic control of heart rate [8, 9]. Studies of the maturation of heart rate control have shown an increasing dominance of parasympathetic control across the first 6 months of life [10]. Preterm birth has been associated with immaturity of autonomic nervous system control of the cardiovascular system. This manifests as higher heart rates [11, 12], reduced heart rate variability [12–14], and decreased baroreflex sensitivity compared to infants born at term [15, 16]. Studies in both preterm [17, 18] and term [8] infants have identified a nadir in basal blood pressure during sleep at 2–4 months of age, when compared to both earlier (2–4 weeks) and later (5–6 months) ages studied; a nadir in physiological anemia also occurs at this age. Blood pressure responses to a cardiovascular challenge (head-up tilting) are also impaired at 2–4 months compared to younger (2–4 weeks) and older (5–6 months) ages [19]. Studies have also shown that there is a maturational reduction in cerebral oxygenation, which is most marked between 2–4 weeks and 2–4 months of age, which may be due to limited or inadequate flow-metabolism coupling at this age [20]. *Thus, 2–4 months of age represents a critical time period when effects of low blood pressure could accentuate decrements in oxygen carrying capacity and delivery to critical organs* [8].

Respiratory control is also immature in the first 6 months of life. In order to maintain blood oxygen levels, adult humans exposed to lowered oxygen levels experience a prompt increase in ventilation that peaks within 3–5 minutes. This period of hyperventilation is sustained for approximately 15–30 minutes before a subsequent decline to prehypoxic baseline values. This response is referred to as the hypoxic ventilatory response (HVR). The HVR in infants is quite different to that of adults. Following exposure to low oxygen levels, infants exhibit a "biphasic" HVR response which typically consists of a transient hyperventilation (within the first 2 minutes) termed the augmented phase, followed by a sustained reduction in ventilation toward or below normoxic levels, termed the depressive phase. This biphasic HVR has been demonstrated in term and preterm infants during both wakefulness and sleep, and studies have observed that the HVR in human infants remains immature up to 2 months after birth [21, 22] and perhaps up to 6 months of age [23].

Infant arousal responses are also affected by postnatal age, although these maturational effects are sleep state-dependent. In infants, two sleep states are defined: quiet sleep (the precursor of non-rapid eye movement [NREM] or deep sleep in adults) and active sleep (the precursor of rapid eye movement [REM] or dreaming sleep). Arousal from sleep can occur spontaneously or as a result of an external (induced) stimulus. Arousal from sleep is a hierarchical process whereby a full cortical arousal is preceded by a sequence of subcortical events, a breathing pause or sigh, a startle, and "thrashing" behavior, with each event stimulating the next in the chain of activation [24]. Previous studies have demonstrated that in response to respiratory (mild hypoxia), tactile (nasal air-jet), and auditory stimulation, total arousability is reduced with increasing age during quiet sleep while remaining unchanged in active sleep [25–27]. Following the introduction of standard scoring criteria for subcortical activation and cortical arousal as separate entities, one study noted that spontaneous subcortical activations decreased with increasing postnatal age, while cortical arousals increased [28]. Conversely, another study analyzed both spontaneous and nasal air-jet induced arousability during supine sleep and found no change in the percentage of cortical arousals (from total responses) throughout the first 6 months of life [29]. Interestingly, when the same infants slept in the prone position, an increased propensity of cortical arousal was identified at 2–4 months, the age when SIDS is most common [29, 30]. This increase in cortical arousals may reflect an innate protective response to ensure an appropriate level of arousal for restoring homeostasis, not only during a vulnerable period of development but also in the presence of an exogenous stressor (e.g., the prone sleeping position).

Arousal and cardiorespiratory responses may also be innately affected, as multiple neuropathologic studies in SIDS victims have supported the concept that SIDS infants are not entirely "normal" prior to death; instead these infants possess some form of underlying vulnerability exposing them to an increased risk for sudden death [31, 32]. The most compelling and reproducible research to date is focused on the hypothesis that SIDS is due to a developmental disorder of medullary serotonergic and related neurotransmitter systems that occurs prenatally but exerts its effects in the postnatal period [33]. The serotonergic system is recognized as a key regulator of the brain's homeostatic control systems, including upper airway control, ventilation and gasping, autonomic control, thermoregulation, chemosensitivity, arousal, and hypoxia-induced plasticity [32, 34]. Recent studies have also identified a significant developmental abnormality of substance P and neurokinin 1 receptor (NK1R) binding in multiple medullary nuclei related to cardiorespiratory function and autonomic control in SIDS cases compared to controls [35]. This research provides support for the hypothesis that there are abnormalities in a multi-neurotransmitter network, with not just one neurotransmitter system involved. Abnormalities have been detected not only in brainstem nuclei that are involved in responses to hypoxia, but also in areas that control head and neck movement. The latter findings may explain why SIDS infants are unable to lift and turn their heads when exposed to a hypoxic situation.

In summary, a large body of work has demonstrated that both autonomic control of the cardiorespiratory system and arousal responses from sleep are maximally affected by the major risk factors for SIDS, at 2–4 months of age when SIDS risk is greatest.

Risk Factors

Why Does Prone Sleeping Increase the Risk?

Prone (stomach) sleeping significantly increases SIDS risk by up to tenfold. Studies have also identified the side sleeping position as a risk factor, most likely because this position is unstable and many infants are found prone after being placed on their side. Infants who are unaccustomed to sleeping prone are particularly at risk if slept in the prone position [36]. Thus, it is important that all caregivers place babies on their back for sleep consistently for each sleep and do not change this routine.

When normal healthy full-term infants sleep in the prone position, several physiological changes ensue in the cardiorespiratory system:

- There is increased peripheral skin temperature and baseline heart rate, lowered blood pressure, and decreased heart rate variability (a measure of autonomic cardiovascular control) [8, 37–45].
- Cerebral oxygenation is reduced and cerebrovascular control impaired [20, 46]; this is exacerbated in preterm born infants [18, 47].
- Cardiac and respiratory responses when arousing from sleep are reduced, when compared to sleeping in the supine position [48, 49].

Importantly, infants who are sleeping in the prone position also have increased total sleep time, particularly time in quiet or deep sleep, with significant reductions in both spontaneous [37, 50–53] and induced arousability to auditory [54] and somatosensory challenges [39, 55, 56]. Hence, parents frequently state that their baby sleeps "better" when placed prone. *However, given that failure to arouse is likely an important contributor to the final pathway to SIDS, parents should be aware that sleeping "better" is not necessarily desirable.*

The prone sleeping position also potentiates the risk of overheating, by reducing the exposed surface area available for radiant heat loss and reducing respiratory heat loss when the infant's face is covered [57]. Infants are less able to maintain adequate respiratory and metabolic homoeostasis when sleeping prone.

Why Do We Advise Avoiding Loose Bedding in the Crib?

The sleeping surface for the baby should be clean, flat, and firm. It is important that the mattress fits snugly in the crib so that the baby cannot become wedged between the mattress and the crib frame. There should be no loose bedding, pillows, crib bumpers, sheepskin, or soft toys that could cover the baby's face. Having the head covered by bedding is a major risk factor, with between 16% and 28% of SIDS infants found with their heads covered. A recent study reported that deaths classified as suffocation were most frequently attributed to soft bedding (69%) [58].

Although a causal relationship with SIDS and head covering has not been established [59, 60], it appears likely that rebreathing and impaired arousal are involved. It has been suggested that the increased SIDS risk associated with head covering may result from hypoxia and hypercapnia via rebreathing of expired air [59, 61]. Head covering with just a sheet in healthy term infants alters autonomic cardiovascular control, increases body temperature [62], and depresses arousal responses in active sleep [63], when compared with no head covering.

What About Swaddling?

Swaddling an infant is often recommended to help the infant settle to sleep in the supine position. Swaddled infants should always be placed supine to sleep, and swaddling should be stopped as soon as infants show any signs of being able to roll. Evidence for this comes from a recent meta-analysis which identified that swaddling risk varied according to position placed for sleep; the risk was highest for prone sleeping (OR, 12.99 [95% CI, 4.14–40.77]), followed by side sleeping (OR, 3.16 [95% CI, 2.08–4.81]) and supine sleeping (OR, 1.93 [95% CI, 1.27–2.93]) [64]. There was evidence to suggest swaddling risk increased with infant age and was associated with a two-fold risk for infants aged >6 months [64].

Studies investigating the effect of swaddling on cardiovascular control are limited. Swaddling elicits a mild increase in respiratory frequency, most likely due to restricted tidal volumes imposed by the firm wrapping [65–67]. No significant effects have been documented on baseline heart rate, skin temperature, or oxygen saturation in term infants when swaddled during sleep [66, 68]. Studies that compared infants who were routinely swaddled to those who were unused to this practice found that sleep time and heart rate variability were only altered in those infants naïve to swaddling [69]. Several studies investigated the effects of swaddling in relation to infant arousability; however, divergent results have been published. The commonly observed decreases in spontaneous movements and startle responses with swaddling are in contrast to effects of other protective factors for SIDS [70, 71]. One study reported that when infants were swaddled, fewer startle responses progressed to a full awakening, indicating an inhibition of the cortical arousal process [72]. More recent studies reported that swaddled infants exhibited increased arousal thresholds (i.e. were harder to arouse) in response to nasal air-jet stimulation. Furthermore, a decreased frequency of full cortical arousals was observed primarily in 3-month-old infants who were unaccustomed to being swaddled [66]. Spontaneous cortical arousals were also decreased in those 3-month-old infants unaccustomed to being swaddled [69]. In contrast to the majority of studies which have shown decreased arousability in swaddled infants, one study found decreased auditory arousal thresholds (i.e. increased arousability) in swaddled infants in active sleep (a state of heightened arousability) when compared to infants who were free to move [68]. Auditory stimuli were not presented in quiet sleep. The study showed decreased arousability during sleep overall and more time spent in quiet sleep as has been demonstrated in other studies. The authors attributed the increased arousability when swaddled to the greater heart rate responses in swaddled conditions [73]. As with the other risk factors discussed above, the mechanisms whereby swaddling may increase the risk for SIDS remain unclear, and further research is required.

Exposure to Cigarette Smoke, Alcohol, and Illicit Drugs Increases the Risk

Prenatal and/or postnatal exposure to cigarette smoke increases infant risk [74, 75], with more than 40 studies showing an increased risk of up to fivefold [76–79]. A recent report using the Centers for Disease Control and Prevention Linked Birth/Infant Death data set (2007–2011) found that smoking more than one cigarette per day doubled the risk of SUID, and that the probability increased linearly with each cigarette smoked, up to 20 cigarettes per day (at which point the incidence plateaued) [80]. Importantly, when mothers quit smoking or reduced their cigarette consumption, their risk was reduced compared to mothers who continued to smoke. The most recent data from the New Zealand SUDI Nationwide Study conducted between 2012 and 2015 found that maternal smoking increased the risk similarly for the indigenous Maori (eightfold) and non-Maori (fivefold) infants [81]. The prevalence of bed-sharing was similar in the two groups, and the study concluded that the main contributor to SUDI was the combination of maternal smoking and bed-sharing.

This increased SIDS risk is likely due to the effects of nicotine exposure on autonomic control and arousal [82–87]. Animal studies have identified that chronic exposure to nicotine in the prenatal period alters serotonergic and nicotinic acetylcholine receptor binding in regions of the medulla; these neurotransmitters are critical to cardiorespiratory control [88]. Studies in infants exposed to maternal smoking have demonstrated altered heart rate and blood pressure control compared with control infants [89–95]. Maternal tobacco smoking also decreases both spontaneous and induced arousability and the proportion of full cortical arousals [30, 55, 96–100]. Newborn infants whose mothers both smoked and used illicit drugs had reduced responses to hypoxia compared to infants whose mothers only smoked cigarettes, and this was most marked when they slept prone, which may explain the increased vulnerability of these infants [101]. Few mothers change their smoking behavior postpartum [102]; therefore it is difficult to ascertain whether these physiological effects are caused by prenatal or postnatal smoke exposure. Environmental smoke (i.e., in the same room) independently increases the risk of SIDS [103, 104]. Importantly, it has been shown that before discharge home from the hospital, preterm infants of smoking mothers already exhibited disruptions in sleep patterns, prior to any postnatal smoke exposure [105].

Exposure to alcohol is also a risk for SIDS [106, 107]. Animal studies have shown that arousal latency to hypoxia is increased when rat pups were exposed to prenatal alcohol [108]. Furthermore, a number of studies have identified that prenatal exposure to illicit drugs also increases the risk for SIDS [109–111], which may be due to impaired responses to hypoxia [112].

In summary, there is considerable evidence from both animal and human studies suggesting that *prenatal exposure to cigarette smoke, alcohol, and illicit drugs have deleterious effects on the developing brain and cardiorespiratory system, particularly with regard to cardiorespiratory control and arousal responses, thus increasing infant vulnerability.* Parents, especially mothers, should be encouraged to reduce smoking as much as possible during pregnancy and after birth and not to allow anyone to smoke around the baby after birth.

Infants Born Preterm Are at an Increased Risk

Maternal smoking may also be a confounding risk factor for SIDS due to its association with other risk factors, such as preterm birth and intrauterine growth restriction (IUGR) [113–116], which likely result from suboptimal intrauterine environments. Regardless of prenatal exposure to maternal smoking, infants born both preterm and IUGR are at increased risk for SIDS [117–125]. The proportion of preterm babies who die suddenly and unexpectedly is approximately four times greater than in full-term infants (20% vs 5%). These proportional differences have remained unchanged since the introduction of public campaigns for reducing the risks [121, 122], despite more than halving the rate for preterm infant deaths attributed to SIDS over the last 20 years [124]. The risk for SIDS in preterm infants is inversely related to gestational age [118, 120, 126–130].

Impaired heart rate control has been reported in term IUGR infants when compared with infants of appropriate size for gestational age [131, 132]. Similarly, preterm infants demonstrate impaired autonomic control compared with term infants studied at, or before, term equivalent age, and this pattern is inversely related to gestational age at birth [11, 12, 133–136]. Longitudinal studies after term equivalent age have identified that preterm infants exhibit lower blood pressure and impaired blood pressure and heart rate control across the first 6 months of corrected age, when compared with age-matched term infants [17, 137–140]. Furthermore, maturation of baroreflex control of blood pressure is affected by gestational age at birth, with infants born very preterm (<32 weeks of gestation) having reduced increases in baroreflex sensitivity compared to both preterm and term infants [141]. Recently, studies have also identified that cerebral oxygenation is also lower in preterm, compared to term, infants across the first 6 months of corrected age [18] and that cerebrovascular control after a head-up tilt is more variable [142], indicating immature or impaired control.

When compared with term infants at matched conceptional ages, preterm infants also exhibit decreased frequencies and durations of spontaneous arousals from sleep [143–145], together with decreased heart rate responses following arousal [146]. Furthermore, preterm infants exhibited longer arousal latencies after exposure to mild hypoxia (15% inspired O_2), reaching significantly lower oxygen saturations, than term infants [147]. Apnea and bradycardia, which are cardiorespiratory conditions commonly associated with prematurity, have also been shown to suppress total arousability when these infants were compared to preterm infants with no history of apnea [148].

In summary, *infants born preterm and/or growth restricted are at increased risk, and alterations in cardiorespiratory control and arousability during sleep likely underpin this vulnerability*. Such physiological disturbances may be further exacerbated during a critical developmental period within infancy and by exposure to exogenous stressors. Thus, it is extremely important that other risk factors, such as prone sleeping and exposure to cigarette smoke, are avoided in preterm infants and that infants are placed supine to sleep as soon as they are medically stable. The American Academy of Pediatrics recommends that they be placed supine from 32 weeks of postmenstrual age [149], so that they and their parents can become used to this position well before discharge from hospital.

Where Should Baby Sleep?

Room-sharing with a baby (without bed-sharing) has been shown to reduce the risk of SIDS by up to 50% [150–158], and it is recommended that babies sleep in their own crib in the parent's bedroom for the first 6–12 months. The protective effect of room-sharing can be partially explained by increased adult supervision and observation of the baby [153, 155, 159–161]. While this does not guarantee the baby's safety, parents/caregivers may become aware of potentially dangerous situations, such as the baby rolling into the prone position or bedclothes covering the face and head [59, 153, 154, 157, 162] or infant distress [157, 159, 160]. Sensory stimulation (e.g., sounds and smells) of the baby through sharing the same room as a parent may also increase arousals from sleep, reduce deep sleep, and support those protective airway mechanisms [158, 159, 163, 164] that are thought to reduce risk.

Bed-Sharing Is a Risk

Bed-sharing has been reported to significantly increase the risk of SIDS, particularly when the mother smokes [80, 152, 156, 157, 165], with more than 50% of SIDS deaths occurring in this situation [166, 167]. Studies have also identified an increased risk with bed-sharing when parents do not smoke [156, 168]. Babies under 3 months of age are at significantly greater risk than older babies [168–170]. These risks include overlaying of the baby by another individual who may be under the influence of alcohol or sedating drugs, entrapment or wedging between the mattress and another object such as a wall, head entrapment in bed railings, and suffocation from pillows and blankets [171–173].

Infants exhibit differences in physiology and behavior when bed-sharing compared to solitary sleeping [174]. When infants from non-smoking families were studied on successive bed-sharing and solitary sleeping nights, bed-sharing was associated with increased awakenings and transient arousals during deep sleep compared to solitary nights [175]. In contrast, another study found that bed-sharing infants spent less time moving and were more likely to have their heads partially or fully covered by bedding than crib-sleeping infants [176]. It is possible that the increased chance of head covering from heavy adult bedding underpins the risk. In summary, the safest place for a baby to sleep is in their own crib in their parent's/caregiver's bedroom for the first 12 months after birth.

Protective Factors

Epidemiologic studies have found that infant care practices such as breastfeeding, dummy/pacifier use, and immunization decrease the risk of SIDS. These potentially protective factors have all been associated with alterations to both cardiovascular autonomic control and arousal responses during sleep. However, results are often inconsistent, and supporting evidence is less extensive than for the risk factors discussed above; thus, the mechanisms for these potentially preventative factors remain controversial among researchers.

Breastfeeding

Breastfeeding reduces the incidence of SIDS by approximately half [177–179]. A recent meta-analysis showed that breastfeeding for at least 2 months was associated with half the risk of SIDS and that breastfeeding does not need to be exclusive to confer this protection [180]. This apparent protection may be a biological effect, given that breastfeeding has been associated with a decreased incidence of diarrhea, vomiting, colds, and other infections; in addition, breast milk is rich in antibodies and many micronutrients [178, 181, 182]. Only one study has assessed the effects of breastfeeding on the cardiovascular system during sleep in term infants, and this study found that heart rate was significantly lower in breast-fed infants when compared with formula-fed infants [183]. Although little is known about the effects of breastfeeding compared to formula feeding on cardiovascular control in infants, physiological studies have demonstrated an apparent promotion of arousal from sleep associated with breastfeeding [184, 185].

Pacifier Use

The protective effect associated with use of a pacifier (also known as a "dummy") has consistently been found in epidemiological studies, with significant associations being described for both usage during the final sleep and "dummy ever used" [152, 168, 186–190]. A likely mechanism for this protective effect is increased heart rate variability, which has been demonstrated during sucking periods in term [191, 192] and preterm infants [193]. In addition, pacifier sucking has been shown to elicit increases in blood pressure in quietly awake or sleeping term infants [192, 194] and in preterm infants [193]. Another potential mechanism for the protective nature of pacifier use is enhanced arousability from sleep. However, results of the few studies that have been conducted are conflicting, with one study reporting decreased arousal thresholds to auditory stimulation observed in infants who regularly used a pacifier, when compared with those who did not use a pacifier [195]. In contrast, other studies have reported no effect of pacifier use on either the frequency or duration of spontaneous arousals in sleeping infants, when studied both with and without a pacifier in the mouth [196, 197]. It has also been hypothesized that sucking on a pacifier during sleep may assist in maintaining airway patency, potentially by a more forward tongue position, thus preventing a pharyngeal vacuum and the consequent sealing of the airway [198, 199]. Although epidemiological studies have provided strong support for pacifier use to be protective, the physiological mechanisms responsible for this protection remain uncertain.

Immunization

The peak incidence of SIDS coincides with the time when infants are receiving their first triple antigen vaccinations. In the 1970s, there were case reports of infant deaths shortly after the diphtheria-tetanus-pertussis immunization, and there were concerns that there was a causal relationship. In 2003, the National Academy of Sciences in the USA reviewed the available data and rejected the idea that there was a causal relationship [200]. Additionally, large population case-control studies have consistently found that immunized infants are less likely to die from SIDS [201–203]. A recent meta-analysis found that the risk of SIDS is halved in immunized infants [204, 205]. There have been limited studies on the physiological benefits of vaccination; however, one study showed that arousal responses and sleep patterns were not affected in the immediate postvaccination period, despite elevated temperature and heart rate [206].

In summary, factors which have been shown to be protective against SIDS show increases in autonomic control and arousability as in the case of dummy/pacifier use and breastfeeding or no change as in the case of immunization.

Summary

- A large number of studies provide physiological evidence that underpins the risk and protective factors associated with sudden infant death during sleep.
- Prone sleeping, maternal smoking, head covering and preterm birth, the major risks for SIDS, decrease arousability from sleep and impair cardiovascular responses.
- Breastfeeding, use of a pacifier, and immunization, known factors associated with a reduced incidence of SIDS, increase or do not alter arousability from sleep and improve autonomic control.
- If parents are made aware of this sound scientific advice as to how their infant's physiology is altered by different infant care practices, then they are more likely to understand the reasons why safe sleeping advice is being recommended.
- Providing safe sleeping advice, which is backed up by sound scientific evidence, is crucial as studies have shown that parents are particularly receptive to advice from their healthcare professional.

References

1. Krous HF, Beckwith JB, Byard RW, Rognum TO, Bajanowski T, Corey T, et al. Sudden infant death syndrome and unclassified sudden infant deaths: a definitional and diagnostic approach. Pediatrics. 2004;114(1):234–8.

2. Filiano J, Kinney HC. A perspective on neuropathologic findings in victims of the sudden infant death syndrome: the triple-risk model. Biol Neonate. 1994;65:194–7.

3. Phillipson EA, Sullivan CE. Arousal: the forgotten response to respiratory stimuli. Am Rev Respir Dis. 1978;118(5):807–9.

4. Horne RSC. Autonomic cardiorespiratory physiology and arousal of the fetus and infant. In: Duncan JR, Byard RW, editors. SIDS sudden infant and early childhood death: the past, the present and the future. Adelaide: University of Adelaide Press; 2018.

5. Gagnon R, Campbell K, Hunse C, Patrick J. Patterns of human fetal heart rate accelerations from 26 weeks to term. Am J Obstet Gynecol. 1987;157:743–8.

6. Karin J, Hirsch M, Akselrod S. An estimate of fetal autonomic state by spectral analysis of fetal heart rate fluctuations. Pediatr Res. 1993;34:134–8.

7. Wakai RT. Assessment of fetal neurodevelopment via fetal magnetocardiography. Exp Neurol. 2004;190:S65–71.

8. Yiallourou SR, Walker AM, Horne RSC. Effects of sleeping position on development of infant cardiovascular control. Arch Dis Child. 2008;93(10):868–72.

9. Harper R, Hoppenbrouwers T, Sterman M, McGinty D, Hodgman J. Polygraphic studies of normal infants during the first six months of life. I. Heart rate and variability as a function of state. Pediatr Res. 1976;10:945–51.

10. Horne RS. Cardio-respiratory control during sleep in infancy. Paediatr Respir Rev. 2014;15(2):163–9.

11. Katona PG, Frasz A, Egbert J. Maturation of cardiac control in full-term and preterm infants during sleep. Early Hum Dev. 1980;4(2):145–59.

12. Eiselt M, Curzi-Dascalova L, Clairambault J, Kauffmann F, Medigue C, Peirano P. Heart rate variability in low-risk prematurely born infants reaching normal term: a comparison with full-term newborns. Early Hum Dev. 1993;32:183–95.

13. de Beer NA, Andriessen P, Berendsen RC, Oei SG, Wijn PF, Oetomo SB. Customized spectral band analysis compared with conventional Fourier analysis of heart rate variability in neonates. Physiol Meas. 2004;25(6):1385–95.

14. Andriessen P, Janssen B, Berendsen RC, Oetomo SB, Wijn PF, Blanco CE. Cardiovascular autonomic regulation in preterm infants: the effect of atropine. Pediatr Res. 2004;56(6):939–46.

15. Waldman S, Krauss AN, Auld PA. Baroreceptors in preterm infants: their relationship to maturity and disease. Dev Med Child Neurol. 1979;21(6):714–22.
16. Gournay V, Drouin E, Roze JC. Development of baroreflex control of heart rate in preterm and full term infants. Arch Dis Child Fetal Neonatal Ed. 2002;86(3):151–4.
17. Witcombe NB, Yiallourou SR, Walker AM, Horne RSC. Blood pressure and heart rate patterns during sleep are altered in preterm-born infants: implications for sudden infant death syndrome. Pediatrics. 2008;122(6):1242–8.
18. Fyfe KL, Yiallourou SR, Wong FY, Odoi A, Walker AM, Horne RS. Cerebral oxygenation in preterm infants. Pediatrics. 2014;134(3):435–45.
19. Yiallourou SR, Walker AM, Horne RSC. Prone sleeping impairs circulatory control during sleep in healthy term infants; implications for sudden infant death syndrome. Sleep. 2008;31(8):1139–46.
20. Wong FY, Witcombe NB, Yiallourou SR, Yorkston S, Dymowski AR, Krishnan L, et al. Cerebral oxygenation is depressed during sleep in healthy term infants when they sleep prone. Pediatrics. 2011;127(3):e558–65.
21. Cohen G, Malcolm G, Henderson-Smart D. Ventilatory response of the newborn infant to mild hypoxia. Pediatr Pulmonol. 1997;24:163–72.
22. Martin RJ, DiFiore JM, Jana L, Davis RL, Miller MJ, Coles SK, et al. Persistence of the biphasic ventilatory response hypoxia in preterm infants. J Pediatr. 1998;132(6):960–4.
23. Parslow PM, Cranage SM, Adamson TM, Harding R, Horne RSC. Arousal and ventilatory responses to hypoxia in sleeping infants: effects of maternal smoking. Respir Physiol Neurobiol. 2004;140:77–87.
24. Lijowska AS, Reed NW, Chiodini BA, Thach BT. Sequential arousal and airway-defensive behavior of infants in asphyxial sleep environments. J Appl Physiol (1985). 1997;83(1):219–28.
25. Parslow PM, Harding R, Cranage SM, Adamson TM, Horne RSC. Ventilatory responses preceding hypoxia-induced arousal in infants: effects of sleep-state. Respir Physiol Neurobiol. 2003;136:235–47.
26. Trinder J, Newman NM, Le Grande M, Whitworth F, Kay A, Pirkis J, et al. Behavioural and EEG responses to auditory stimuli during sleep in newborn infants and in infants aged 3 months. Biol Psychol. 1990;90:213–27.

27. Parslow PM, Harding R, Cranage SM, Adamson TM, Horne RSC. Arousal responses to somatosensory and mild hypoxic stimuli are depressed during quiet sleep in healthy term infants. Sleep. 2003;26(6):739–44.

28. Montemitro E, Franco P, Scaillet S, Kato I, Groswasser J, Villa MP, et al. Maturation of spontaneous arousals in healthy infants. Sleep. 2008;31(1):47–54.

29. Richardson HL, Walker AM, Horne RSC. Sleep position alters arousal processes maximally at the high-risk age for sudden infant death syndrome. J Sleep Res. 2008;17:450–7.

30. Richardson HL, Walker AM, Horne RSC. Maternal smoking impairs arousal patterns in sleeping infants. Sleep. 2009;32(4):515–21.

31. Harper RM, Kinney HC. Potential mechanisms of failure in the sudden infant death syndrome. Curr Pediatr Rev. 2010;6(1):39–47.

32. Kinney HC, Thach BT. The sudden infant death syndrome. N Engl J Med. 2009;361(8):795–805.

33. Bright FM, Vink R, Byard RW. Brainstem neuropathology in sudden infant death syndrome. In: Duncan JR, Byard RW, editors. SIDS sudden infant and early childhood death: the past, the present and the future. Adelaide: University of Adelaide Press; 2018.

34. Kinney HC, Richerson GB, Dymecki SM, Darnall RA, Nattie EE. The brainstem and serotonin in the sudden infant death syndrome. Annu Rev Pathol. 2009;4:517–50.

35. Bright FM, Vink R, Byard RW. The potential role of substance P in brainstem homeostatic control in the pathogenesis of sudden infant death syndrome (SIDS). Neuropeptides. 2018;70:1–8.

36. Li DK, Petitti DB, Willinger M, McMahon R, Odouli R, Vu H, et al. Infant sleeping position and the risk of sudden infant death syndrome in California, 1997–2000. Am J Epidemiol. 2003;157(5):446–55.

37. Galland BC, Reeves G, Taylor BJ, Bolton DP. Sleep position, autonomic function, and arousal. Arch Dis Child Fetal Neonatal Ed. 1998;78(3):F189–94.

38. Galland BC, Taylor BJ, Bolton DP, Sayers RM. Vasoconstriction following spontaneous sighs and head-up tilts in infants sleeping prone and supine. Early Hum Dev. 2000;58(2):119–32.

39. Horne R, Ferens D, Watts A, Vitkovic J, Lacey B, Andrew S, et al. The prone sleeping position impairs arousability in term infants. J Pediatr. 2001;138:811–6.

40. Ariagno RL, Mirmiran M, Adams MM, Saporito AG, Dubin AM, Baldwin RB. Effect of position on sleep, heart rate variability, and QT interval in preterm infants at 1 and 3 months' corrected age. Pediatrics. 2003;111:622–5.

41. Sahni R, Schulz H, Kashyap S, Ohira-Kist K, Fifer WP, Myers MM. Postural differences in cardiac dynamics during quiet and active sleep in low birthweight infants. Acta Paediatr. 1999;88:1396–401.

42. Gabai N, Cohen A, Mahagney A, Bader D, Tirosh E. Arterial blood flow and autonomic function in full-term infants. Clin Physiol Funct Imaging. 2006;26:127–31.

43. Kahn A, Groswasser J, Sottiaux M, Rebuffat E, Franco P, Dramaix M. Prone or supine body position and sleep characteristics in infants. Pediatrics. 1993;91(6):1112–5.

44. Chong A, Murphy N, Matthews T. Effect of prone sleeping on circulatory control in infants. Arch Dis Child. 2000;82:253–6.

45. Ammari A, Schulze KF, Ohira-Kist K, Kashyap S, Fifer WP, Myers MM, et al. Effects of body position on thermal, cardiorespiratory and metabolic activity in low birth weight infants. Early Hum Dev. 2009;85:497–501.

46. Wong F, Yiallourou SR, Odoi A, Browne P, Walker AM, Horne RS. Cerebrovascular control is altered in healthy term infants when they sleep prone. Sleep. 2013;36(12):1911–8.

47. Fyfe KL, Yiallourou SR, Wong FY, Horne RS. The development of cardiovascular and cerebral vascular control in preterm infants. Sleep Med Rev. 2014;18(4):299–310.

48. Franco P, Grosswasser J, Sottiaux M, Broadfield E, Kahn A. Decreased cardiac responses to auditory stimulation during prone sleep. Pediatrics. 1996;97:174–8.

49. Tuladhar R, Harding R, Cranage SM, Adamson TM, Horne RSC. Effects of sleep position, sleep state and age on heart rate responses following provoked arousal in term infants. Early Hum Dev. 2003;71:157–69.

50. Ariagno R, van Liempt S, Mirmiran M. Fewer spontaneous arousals during prone sleep in preterm infants at 1 and 3 months corrected age. J Perinatol. 2006;26:306–12.

51. Goto K, Maeda T, Mirmiran M, Ariagno R. Effects of prone and supine position on sleep characteristics in preterm infants. Psychiatry Clin Neurosci. 1999;53:315–7.

52. Bhat RY, Hannam S, Pressler R, Rafferty GF, Peacock JL, Greenough A. Effect of prone and supine position on sleep, apneas, and arousal in preterm infants. Pediatrics. 2006;118:101–7.

53. Kato I, Scaillet S, Groswasser J, Montemitro E, Togari H, Lin J, et al. Spontaneous arousability in prone and supine position in healthy infants. Sleep. 2006;29(6):785–90.

54. Franco P, Pardou A, Hassid S, Lurquin P, Groswasser J, Kahn A. Auditory arousal thresholds are higher when infants sleep in the prone position. J Pediatr. 1998;132:240–3.

55. Horne RSC, Ferens D, Watts A-M, Vitkovic J, Andrew S, Cranage SM, et al. Effects of maternal tobacco smoking, sleeping position and sleep state on arousal in healthy term infants. Arch Dis Child Fetal Neonatal Ed. 2002;87:F100–F5.

56. Horne RSC, Bandopadhayay P, Vitkovic J, Cranage SM, Adamson TM. Effects of age and sleeping position on arousal from sleep in preterm infants. Sleep. 2002;25:746–50.

57. Ponsonby A, Dwyer T, Gibbons LE, Cochrane JA, Jones ME, McCall MJ. Thermal environment and sudden infant death syndrome: case-control study. BMJ. 1992;304:279–91.

58. Erck Lambert AB, Parks SE, Cottengim C, Faulkner M, Hauck FR, Shapiro-Mendoza CK. Sleep-related infant suffocation deaths attributable to soft bedding, overlay, and wedging. Pediatrics. 2019;143(5):e20183408.

59. Blair PS, Mitchell EA, Heckstall-Smith EMA, Fleming PJ. Head covering a major modifiable risk factor for sudden infant death syndrome: a systematic review. Arch Dis Child. 2008;93(9):778–83.

60. Mitchell EA, Thompson JM, Becroft DM, Bajanowski T, Brinkmann B, Happe A, et al. Head covering and the risk for SIDS: findings from the New Zealand and German SIDS case-control studies. Pediatrics. 2008;121(6):e1478–e83.

61. Paluszynska DA, Harris KA, Thach BT. Influence of sleep position experience on ability of prone-sleeping infants to escape from asphyxiating microenvironments by changing head position. Pediatrics. 2004;114(6):1634–9.

62. Franco P, Lipshut W, Valente F, Adams M, Grosswasser J, Kahn A. Cardiac autonomic characteristics in infants sleeping with their head covered by bedclothes. J Sleep Res. 2003;12(2):125–32.

63. Franco P, Lipshutz W, Valente F, Adams S, Scaillet S, Kahn A. Decreased arousals in infants who sleep with the face covered by bedclothes. Pediatrics. 2002;109(6):1112–7.

64. Pease AS, Fleming PJ, Hauck FR, Moon RY, Horne RS, L'Hoir MP, et al. Swaddling and the risk of sudden infant death syndrome: a meta-analysis. Pediatrics. 2016;137(6):e20153275.

65. Gerard CM, Harris KA, Thach BT. Physiologic studies on swaddling: an ancient child care practice, which may promote the supine position for infant sleep. J Pediatr. 2002;141(3):398–403.
66. Richardson HL, Walker AM, Horne RSC. Minimizing the risk of sudden infant death syndrome: to swaddle or not to swaddle? J Pediatr. 2009;155(4):475–81; ePub August 2009.
67. Narangerel G, Pollock J, Manaseki-Holland S, Henderson J. The effects of swaddling on oxygen saturation and respiratory rate of healthy infants in Mongolia. Acta Paediatr. 2007;96:261–5.
68. Franco P, Seret N, Van Hees J, Scaillet S, Grosswasser J, Kahn A. Influence of swaddling on sleep and arousal characteristics of healthy infants. Pediatrics. 2005;115:1307–11.
69. Richardson HL, Walker AM, Horne RS. Influence of swaddling experience on spontaneous arousal patterns and autonomic control in sleeping infants. J Pediatr. 2010;157(1):85–91.
70. Lipton EL, Steinschneider A, Richmond JB. Swaddling, a child care practice: historical, cultural, and experimental observations. Pediatrics. 1965;35(3P2):521–67.
71. Chisholm JS. Swaddling, cradleboards and the development of children. Early Hum Dev. 1978;2(3):255–75.
72. Gerard CM, Harris KA, Thach BT. Spontaneous arousals in supine infants while swaddled and unswaddled during rapid eye movement and quiet sleep. Pediatrics. 2002;110(6):70–6.
73. Franco P, Scaillet S, Grosswasser J, Kahn A. Increased cardiac autonomic responses to auditory challenges in swaddled infants. Sleep. 2004;27(8):1527–32.
74. Mitchell E, Scragg R, Stewart AW, Becroft DMO, Taylor B, Ford RPK, et al. Results from the first year of the New Zealand cot death study. N Z Med J. 1991;104:71–6.
75. Matturri L, Ottaviani G, Lavezzi AM. Maternal smoking and sudden infant death syndrome: epidemiological study related to pathology. Virchows Arch. 2006;449:697–706.
76. Anderson HR, Cook DG. Passive smoking and sudden infant death syndrome: review of the epidemilogical evidence. Thorax. 1997;52:1003–9.
77. Blair PS, Bensley D, Smith I, Bacon C, Taylor B, Berry J. Smoking and the sudden infant death syndrome: results from 1993-5 case-control study for confidential inquiry into stillbirths and deaths in infancy. BMJ. 1996;313:195–8.
78. Dwyer T, Ponsonby A, Couper D. Tobacco smoke exposure at one month of age and subsequent risk of SIDS – a prospective study. Am J Epidemiol. 1999;149:593–602.

79. Haglund B. Cigarette smoking and sudden infant death syndrome: some salient points in the debate. Acta Paediatr Suppl. 1993;389:37–9.

80. Anderson TM, Lavista Ferres JM, Ren SY, Moon RY, Goldstein RD, Ramirez JM, et al. Maternal smoking before and during pregnancy and the risk of sudden unexpected infant death. Pediatrics. 2019;143(4):e20183325.

81. MacFarlane M, Thompson JMD, Zuccollo J, McDonald G, Elder D, Stewart AW, et al. Smoking in pregnancy is a key factor for sudden infant death among Maori. Acta Paediatr. 2018;107(11):1924–31.

82. Machaalani R, Say M, Waters KA. Effects of cigarette smoke exposure on nicotinic acetylcholine receptor subunits alpha7 and beta2 in the sudden infant death syndrome (SIDS) brainstem. Toxicol Appl Pharmacol. 2011;257(3):396–404.

83. Machaalani R, Ghazavi E, Hinton T, Waters KA, Hennessy A. Cigarette smoking during pregnancy regulates the expression of specific nicotinic acetylcholine receptor (nAChR) subunits in the human placenta. Toxicol Appl Pharmacol. 2014;276(3):204–12.

84. Machaalani R, Waters KA. Neurochemical abnormalities in the brainstem of the sudden infant death syndrome (SIDS). Paediatr Respir Rev. 2014;15(4):293–300.

85. Lavezzi AM, Mecchia D, Matturri L. Neuropathology of the area postrema in sudden intrauterine and infant death syndromes related to tobacco smoke exposure. Auton Neurosci. 2012;166(1–2):29–34.

86. Hunt NJ, Russell B, Du MK, Waters KA, Machaalani R. Changes in orexinergic immunoreactivity of the piglet hypothalamus and pons after exposure to chronic postnatal nicotine and intermittent hypercapnic hypoxia. Eur J Neurosci. 2016;43(12):1612–22.

87. Vivekanandarajah A, Chan YL, Chen H, Machaalani R. Prenatal cigarette smoke exposure effects on apoptotic and nicotinic acetylcholine receptor expression in the infant mouse brainstem. Neurotoxicology. 2016;53:53–63.

88. Duncan JR, Garland M, Myers MM, Fifer WP, Yang M, Kinney HC, et al. Prenatal nicotine-exposure alters fetal autonomic activity and medullary neurotransmitter receptors: implications for sudden infant death syndrome. J Appl Physiol. 2009;107(5):1579–90.

89. Browne CA, Colditz PB, Dunster KR. Infant autonomic function is altered by maternal smoking during pregnancy. Early Hum Dev. 2000;59:209–18.

90. Dahlstrom A, Ebersjo C, Lundell B. Nicotine in breast milk influences heart rate variability in the infant. Acta Paediatr. 2008;97(8):1075–9.

91. Fifer WP, Fingers ST, Youngman M, Gomez-Gribben E, Myers MM. Effects of alcohol and smoking during pregnancy on infant autonomic control. Dev Psychobiol. 2009;51:234–42.

92. Cohen G, Vella S, Jeffery H, Lagercrantz H, Katz-Salamon M. Cardiovascular stress hyperreactivity in babies of smokers and in babies born preterm. Circulation. 2008;118(18):1848–53.

93. Thiriez G, Bouhaddi M, Mourot L, Nobili F, Fortrat JO, Menget A, et al. Heart rate variability in preterm infants and maternal smoking during pregnancy. Clin Auton Res. 2009;19(3):149–56.

94. Viskari-Lahdeoja S, Hytinantti T, Andersson S, Kirjavainen T. Heart rate and blood pressure control in infants exposed to maternal cigarette smoking. Acta Paediatr. 2008;97(11):1535–41.

95. Franco P, Chabanski S, Szliwowski H, Dramaix M, Kahn A. Influence of maternal smoking on autonomic nervous system in healthy infants. Pediatr Res. 2000;47(2):215–20.

96. Sawnani H, Jackson T, Murphy T, Beckerman R, Simakajornboon N. The effect of maternal smoking on respiratory and arousal patterns in preterm infants during sleep. Am J Respir Crit Care Med. 2004;169:733–8.

97. Tirosh E, Libon D, Bader D. The effect of maternal smoking during pregnancy on sleep respiratory and arousal patterns in neonates. J Perinatol. 1996;16(6):435–8.

98. Franco P, Groswasser J, Hassid S, Lanquart J, Scaillet S, Kahn A. Prenatal exposure to cigarette smoking is associated with a decrease in arousal in infants. J Pediatr. 1999;135(1):34–8.

99. Chang AB, Wilson SJ, Masters IB, Yuill M, Williams G, Hubbard M. Altered arousal response in infants exposed to cigarette smoke. Arch Dis Child. 2003;88:30–3.

100. Lewis KW, Bosque EM. Deficient hypoxia awakening response in infants of smoking mothers: possible relationship to sudden infant death syndrome. J Pediatr. 1995;127(5):691–9.

101. Rossor T, Ali K, Bhat R, Trenear R, Rafferty G, Greenough A. The effects of sleeping position, maternal smoking and substance misuse on the ventilatory response to hypoxia in the newborn period. Pediatr Res. 2018;84(3):411–8.

102. Johansson A, Halling A, Hermansson G. Indoor and outdoor smoking. Impact on children's health. Eur J Pub Health. 2003;13(1):61–6.

103. Schoendorf KC, Kiely JL. Relationship of sudden infant death syndrome to maternal smoking during and after pregnancy. Pediatrics. 1992;90(6):905–8.

104. Klonoff-Cohen HS, Edelstein SL, Lefkowitz ES, Srinivasan IP, Kaegi D, Chang JC, et al. The effect of passive smoking and tobacco exposure through breast milk on sudden infant death syndrome. JAMA. 1995;273(10):795–8.

105. Stephan-Blanchard E, Telliez F, Leke A, Djeddi D, Bach V, Libert J, et al. The influence of in utero exposure to smoking on sleep patterns in preterm neonates. Sleep. 2008;31(12):1683–9.

106. Strandberg-Larsen K, Gronboek M, Andersen AM, Andersen PK, Olsen J. Alcohol drinking pattern during pregnancy and risk of infant mortality. Epidemiology. 2009;20(6):884–91.

107. O'Leary CM, Jacoby PJ, Bartu A, D'Antoine H, Bower C. Maternal alcohol use and sudden infant death syndrome and infant mortality excluding SIDS. Pediatrics. 2013;131(3):e770–8.

108. Sirieix CM, Tobia CM, Schneider RW, Darnall RA. Impaired arousal in rat pups with prenatal alcohol exposure is modulated by GABAergic mechanisms. Physiol Rep. 2015;3(6):e12424.

109. Rajegowda BK, Kandall SR, Falciglia H. Sudden unexpected death in infants of narcotic-dependent mothers. Early Hum Dev. 1978;2(3):219–25.

110. Chavez CJ, Ostrea EM Jr, Stryker JC, Smialek Z. Sudden infant death syndrome among infants of drug-dependent mothers. J Pediatr. 1979;95(3):407–9.

111. Williams SM, Mitchell EA, Taylor BJ. Are risk factors for sudden infant death syndrome different at night? Arch Dis Child. 2002;87(4):274–8.

112. Ali K, Rossor T, Bhat R, Wolff K, Hannam S, Rafferty GF, et al. Antenatal substance misuse and smoking and newborn hypoxic challenge response. Arch Dis Child Fetal Neonatal Ed. 2016;101(2):F143–8.

113. Andriessen P, Koolen AMP, Berendsen RCM, Wijn PFF, ten Broeke EDM, Oei SG, et al. Cardiovascular fluctuations and transfer function analysis in stable preterm infants. Pediatr Res. 2003;53(1):89–97.

114. Mitchell EA, Ford RPK, Stewart AW, Taylor BJ, Becroft DMO, Thompson JMD, et al. Smoking and the sudden infant death syndrome. Pediatrics. 1993;91:893–6.

115. Brooke H, Gibson A, Tappin D, Brown H. Case control study of sudden infant death syndrome in Scotland, 1992–5. BMJ. 1997;314:1516–20.
116. Schellscheidt J, Oyen N, Jorch G. Interactions between maternal smoking and other perinatal risk factors for SIDS. Acta Paediatr. 1997;86:857–63.
117. Bergman AB, Ray CG, Pomeroy MA, Wahl PW, Beckwith JB. Studies of the sudden infant death syndrome in King County, Washington. 3. Epidemiology. Pediatrics. 1972;49(6):860–70.
118. Grether JK, Schulman J. Sudden infant death syndrome and birth weight. J Pediatr. 1989;114:561–7.
119. Adams MM, Rhodes PH, McCarthy BJ. Are race and length of gestation related to age at death in the sudden infant death syndrome? Paediatr Perinat Epidemiol. 1990;4(3):325–39.
120. Malloy MH, Hoffman HJ. Prematurity, sudden infant death syndrome, and age of death. Pediatrics. 1995;96(3):464–71.
121. Blair PS, Platt MW, Smith IJ, Fleming PJ, CESDI SUDI Research Group. Sudden infant death syndrome and sleeping position in pre-term and low birth weight infants: an opportunity for targeted intervention. Arch Dis Child. 2006;91:101–6.
122. Thompson JM, Mitchell EA, New Zealand Cot Death Study Group. Are the risk factors for SIDS different for preterm and term infants? Arch Dis Child. 2006;91(2):107–11.
123. Gilbert NL, Fell DB, Joseph KS, Liu S, Leon JA, Sauve R, et al. Temporal trends in sudden infant death syndrome in Canada from 1991 to 2005: contribution of changes in cause of death assignment practices and in maternal and infant characteristics. Paediatr Perinat Epidemiol. 2012;26(2):124–30.
124. Malloy MH. Prematurity and sudden infant death syndrome: United States 2005–2007. J Perinatol. 2013;33(6):470–5.
125. Ostfeld BM, Schwartz-Soicher O, Reichman NE, Teitler JO, Hegyi T. Prematurity and sudden unexpected infant deaths in the United States. Pediatrics. 2017;140(1):e20163334.
126. Peterson DR. Sudden, unexpected death in infants. An epidemiologic study. Am J Epidemiol. 1966;84(3):478–82.
127. Standfast SJ, Jereb S, Janerich DT. The epidemiology of sudden infant death in upstate New York. J Am Med Assoc. 1979;241(11):1121–4.
128. Hoffman HJ, Damus K, Hillman L, Krongrad E. Risk factors for SIDS: results of the National Institute of Child Health and Human Development SIDS cooperative epidemiology study. Ann N Y Acad Sci. 1988;533:13–30.

42   R. S. C. Horne

129. Hoffman HJ, Hillman LS. Epidemiology of the sudden infant death syndrome: maternal , neonatal, and postneonatal risk factors. Clin Perinatol. 1992;19(4):717–37.
130. Malloy MH, Freeman DH Jr. Birth weight- and gestational age-specific sudden infant death syndrome mortality: United States, 1991 versus 1995. Pediatrics. 2000;105(6):1227–31.
131. Galland BC, Taylor B, Bolton DPG, Sayers RM. Heart rate variability and cardiac reflexes in small for gestational age infants. J Appl Physiol. 2006;100(3):933–9.
132. Spassov L, Curzi-Dascalova L, Clairambault J, Kauffmann F, Eiselt M, Medigue C, et al. Heart rate and heart rate variability during sleep in small-for-gestational age newborns. Pediatr Res. 1994;35(4 Pt 1):500–5.
133. Eiselt M, Zwiener U, Witte H, Curzi-Dascalova L. Influence of prematurity and extrauterine development on the sleep state dependant heart rate patterns. Somnologie. 2002;6(3):116–23.
134. Patural H, Barthelemy JC, Pichot V, Mazzocchi C, Teyssier G, Damon G, et al. Birth prematurity determines prolonged autonomic nervous system immaturity. Clin Auton Res. 2004;14:391–5.
135. Patural H, Pichot V, Jaziri F, Teyssier G, Gaspoz JM, Roche F, et al. Autonomic cardiac control of very preterm newborns: a prolonged dysfunction. Early Hum Dev. 2008;84(10):681–7.
136. Longin E, Gerstner T, Schaible T, Lanz T, Konig S. Maturation of the autonomic nervous system: differences in heart rate variability in premature vs. term infants. J Perinat Med. 2006;34:303–8.
137. Witcombe NB, Yiallourou SR, Sands SA, Walker AM, Horne RS. Preterm birth alters the maturation of baroreflex sensitivity in sleeping infants. Pediatrics. 2012;129(1):e89–96.
138. Witcombe NB, Yiallourou SR, Walker AM, Horne RSC. Delayed blood pressure recovery after head-up tilting during sleep in preterm infants. J Sleep Res. 2010;19:93–102.
139. Fyfe KL, Yiallourou SR, Wong FY, Odoi A, Walker AM, Horne RS. The effect of gestational age at birth on post-term maturation of heart rate variability. Sleep. 2015;38(10):1635–44.
140. Yiallourou SR, Witcombe NB, Sands SA, Walker AM, Horne RS. The development of autonomic cardiovascular control is altered by preterm birth. Early Hum Dev. 2013;89(3):145–52.

141. Fyfe KL, Yiallourou SR, Wong FY, Odoi A, Walker AM, Horne RS. Gestational age at birth affects maturation of baroreflex control. J Pediatr. 2015;166(3):559–65.

142. Fyfe K, Odoi A, Yiallourou SR, Wong F, Walker AM, Horne RS. Preterm infants exhibit greater variability in cerebrovascular control than term infants. Sleep. 2015;38(9):1411–21.

143. Horne RSC, Cranage SM, Chau B, Adamson TM. Effects of prematurity on arousal from sleep in the newborn infant. Pediatr Res. 2000;47:468–74.

144. Scher MS, Steppe DA, Dahl RE, Asthana S, Guthrie RD. Comparison of EEG sleep measures in healthy full-term and preterm infants at matched conceptional ages. Sleep. 1992;15(5):442–8.

145. Richardson HL, Horne RS. Arousal from sleep pathways are affected by the prone sleeping position and preterm birth: preterm birth, prone sleeping and arousal from sleep. Early Hum Dev. 2013;89(9):705–11.

146. Tuladhar R, Harding R, Adamson TM, Horne RSC. Comparison of postnatal development of heart rate responses to trigeminal stimulation in sleeping preterm and term infants. J Sleep Res. 2005;14:29–36.

147. Verbeek MMA, Richardson HL, Parslow PM, Walker AM, Harding R, Horne RSC. Arousal and ventilatory responses to mild hypoxia in sleeping preterm infants. J Sleep Res. 2008;17:344–53.

148. Horne RSC, Andrew S, Mitchell K, Sly DJ, Cranage SM, Chau B, et al. Apnoea of prematurity and arousal from sleep. Early Hum Dev. 2001;61:119–33.

149. American Academy of Pediatrics, Committee on Fetus and Newborn. Hospital discharge of the high-risk neonate. Pediatrics. 2008;122(5):1119–26.

150. Mitchell EA, Thompson JMD. Co-sleeping increases the risk of SIDS, but sleeping in the parents' bedroom lowers it. In: Rognum TO, editor. Sudden infant death syndrome: new trends in the nineties. Oslo: Scandinavian University Press; 1995. p. 266–9.

151. Blair PS, Fleming PJ, Smith IJ, Platt MW, Young J, Nadin P, et al. Babies sleeping with parents: case-control study of factors influencing the risk of the sudden infant death syndrome. CESDI SUDI Research Group. BMJ (Clinical Research Ed). 1999;319(7223):1457–61.

152. Carpenter RG, Irgens LM, Blair PS, England PD, Fleming P, Huber J, et al. Sudden unexplained infant death in 20 regions in Europe: case control study. Lancet (London, England). 2004;363(9404):185–91.

153. Blair PS, Platt MW, Smith IJ, Fleming PJ, SESDI SUDI Research Group. Sudden infant death syndrome and the time of death: factors associated with night-time and day-time deaths. Int J Epidemiol. 2006;35(6):1563–9.

154. Kuhnert R, Schlaud M, Poethko-Muller C, Vennemann M, Fleming P, Blair PS, et al. Reanalyses of case-control studies examining the temporal association between sudden infant death syndrome and vaccination. Vaccine. 2012;30(13):2349–56.

155. American Academy of Pediatrics: Task Force on Sudden Infant Death Syndrome. SIDS and other sleep-related infant deaths: updated 2016 recommendations for a safe infant sleeping environment. Pediatrics. 2016;138(5):e20162938.

156. Carpenter R, McGarvey C, Mitchell EA, Tappin DM, Vennemann MM, Smuk M, et al. Bed sharing when parents do not smoke: is there a risk of SIDS? An individual level analysis of five major case-control studies. BMJ Open. 2013;3(5):e002299.

157. Blair PS, Sidebotham P, Pease A, Fleming PJ. Bed-sharing in the absence of hazardous circumstances: is there a risk of sudden infant death syndrome? An analysis from two case-control studies conducted in the UK. PLoS One. 2014;9(9):e107799.

158. Horne RSC, Hauck FR, Moon RY. Sudden infant death syndrome and advice for safe sleeping. BMJ. 2015;350:h1989.

159. McKenna JJ, McDade T. Why babies should never sleep alone: a review of the co-sleeping controversy in relation to SIDS, bedsharing and breast feeding. Paediatr Respir Rev. 2005;6(2):134–52.

160. Scragg RK, Mitchell EA, Stewart AW, Ford RP, Taylor BJ, Hassall IB, et al. Infant room-sharing and prone sleep position in sudden infant death syndrome. New Zealand Cot Death Study Group. Lancet (London, England). 1996;347(8993): 7–12.

161. Blair PS, Ball HL. The prevalence and characteristics associated with parent-infant bed-sharing in England. Arch Dis Child. 2004;89(12):1106–10.

162. Ball HL, Moya E, Fairley L, Westman J, Oddie S, Wright J. Infant care practices related to sudden infant death syndrome

in South Asian and White British families in the UK. Paediatr Perinat Epidemiol. 2012;26(1):3–12.

163. Mosko S, Richard C, McKenna J. Maternal sleep and arousals during bedsharing with infants. Sleep. 1997;20(2):142–50.

164. Simard V, Lara-Carrasco J, Paquette T, Nielsen T. Breastfeeding, maternal depressive mood and roomsharing as predictors of sleep fragmentation in 12-week old infants: a longitudinal study. Early Child Dev Care. 2011;181(8):1063–77.

165. Blair PS, Sidebotham P, Evason-Coombe C, Edmonds M, Heckstall-Smith EM, Fleming P. Hazardous cosleeping environments and risk factors amenable to change: case-control study of SIDS in south west England. BMJ. 2009;339:b3666.

166. Escott AS, Elder ED, Zuccollo JM. Sudden unexpected infant death and bedsharing: referrals to the Wellington Coroner 1997-2006. N Z Med J. 2009;122(1298):59–68.

167. Hauck FR, Signore C, Fein SB, Raju TNK. Infant sleeping arrangements and practices during the first year of life. Pediatrics. 2008;122:S113–S20.

168. Vennemann MM, Bajanowski T, Brinkmann B, Jorch G, Sauerland C, Mitchell EA, et al. Sleep environment risk factors for sudden infant death syndrome: the German sudden infant death syndrome study. Pediatrics. 2009;123(4):1162–70.

169. Tappin D, Ecob R, Brooke H. Bedsharing, roomsharing, and sudden infant death syndrome in Scotland: a case-control study. J Pediatr. 2005;147(1):32–7.

170. McGarvey C, McDonnell M, Chong A, O'Regan M, Matthews T. Factors relating to the infant's last sleep environment in sudden infant death syndrome in the Republic of Ireland. Arch Dis Child. 2003;88(12):1058–64.

171. Collins KA. Death by overlaying and wedging: a 15-year retrospective study. Am J Forensic Med Pathol. 2001;22(2):155–9.

172. Kemp JS, Unger B, Wilkins D, Psara RM, Ledbetter TL, Graham MA, et al. Unsafe sleep practices and an analysis of bedsharing among infants dying suddenly and unexpectedly: results of a four-year, population-based, death-scene investigation study of sudden infant death syndrome and related deaths. Pediatrics. 2000;106(3):E41.

173. Nakamura S, Wind M, Danello MA. Review of hazards associated with children placed in adult beds. Arch Pediatr Adolesc Med. 1999;153(10):1019–23.

174. Baddock SA, Purnell MT, Blair PS, Pease AS, Elder DE, Galland BC. The influence of bed-sharing on infant physiology,

breastfeeding and behaviour: a systematic review. Sleep Med Rev. 2019;43:106–17.

175. McKenna JJ, Mosko SS. Sleep and arousal synchrony and independence among mothers and infants sleeping apart and together (same bed): an experiment in evolutionary medicine. Acta Paediatr Suppl. 1994;397:94–102.

176. Baddock SA, Galland BC, Bolton DP, Williams SM, Taylor BJ. Differences in infant and parent behaviors during routine bed sharing compared with cot sleeping in the home setting. Pediatrics. 2006;117(5):1599–607.

177. Vennemann MM, Bajanowski T, Brinkmann B, Jorch G, Yucsesan K, Sauerland C, et al. Does breastfeeding reduce the risk of sudden infant death syndrome? Pediatrics. 2009;123(3):e406–e10.

178. Hoffman HJ, Damus K, Hillman L, Krongrad E. Risk factors for SIDS. Results of the National Institute of Child Health and Human Development SIDS Cooperative Epidemiological Study. Ann N Y Acad Sci. 1988;533:13–30.

179. Hauck FR, Thompson JM, Tanabe KO, Moon RY, Vennemann MM. Breastfeeding and reduced risk of sudden infant death syndrome: a meta-analysis. Pediatrics. 2011;128(1):103–10.

180. Thompson JMD, Tanabe K, Moon RY, Mitchell EA, McGarvey C, Tappin D, et al. Duration of breastfeeding and risk of SIDS: an individual participant data meta-analysis. Pediatrics. 2017;140(5):e20171324.

181. Gordon AE, Saadi AT, MacKenzie DAC, Molony N, James VS, Weir DM, et al. The protective eject of breast feeding in relation to sudden infant death syndrome (SIDS): III. Detection of IgA antibodies in human milk that bind to bacterial toxins implicated in SIDS. FEMS Immunol Med Microbiol. 1999;25(1–2):175–82.

182. McVea KLSP, Turner PD, Peppler DK. The role of breastfeeding in sudden infant death syndrome. J Hum Lact. 2000;16(1):13–20.

183. Butte NF, Smith EO, Garza C. Heart rate of breast-fed and formula-fed infants. J Pediatr Gastroenterol Nutr. 1991;13(4):391–6.

184. Elias MF, Nicolson NA, Bora C, Johnston J. Sleep/wake patterns of breast-fed infants in the first 2 years of life. Pediatrics. 1986;77(3):322–9.

185. Horne RS, Parslow PM, Ferens D, Watts AM, Adamson TM. Comparison of evoked arousability in breast and formula fed infants. Arch Dis Child. 2004;89(1):22–5.

186. Fleming PJ, Blair PS, Pollard K, Platt MW, Leach C, Smith I, et al. Pacifier use and sudden infant death syndrome: results from the CESDI/SUDI case control study. CESDI SUDI Research Team. Arch Dis Child. 1999;81(2):112–6.

187. Hauck FR, Omojokun OO, Siadaty MS. Do pacifiers reduce the risk of sudden infant death syndrome? A meta-analysis. Pediatrics. 2005;116(5):e716–23.

188. Li DK, Willinger M, Petitti DB, Odouli R, Liu L, Hoffman HJ. Use of a dummy (pacifier) during sleep and risk of sudden infant death syndrome (SIDS): population based case-control study. BMJ. 2006;332(7532):18–22.

189. Mitchell EA, Blair PS, L'Hoir MP. Should pacifiers be recommended to prevent sudden infant death syndrome? Pediatrics. 2006;117(5):1755–8.

190. Horne RS, Hauck FR, Moon RY, L'Hoir MP, Blair PS, Physiology and Epidemiology Working Groups of the International Society for the Study and Prevention of Perinatal and Infant Death. Dummy (pacifier) use and sudden infant death syndrome: potential advantages and disadvantages. J Paediatr Child Health. 2014;50(3):170–4.

191. Franco P, Chabanski S, Scaillet S, Grosswasser J, Kahn A. Pacifier use modifies infant's cardiac autonomic controls during sleep. Early Hum Dev. 2004;77:99–108.

192. Yiallourou SR, Poole H, Prathivadi P, Odoi A, Wong FY, Horne RS. The effects of dummy/pacifier use on infant blood pressure and autonomic activity during sleep. Sleep Med. 2014;15(12):1508–16.

193. Horne RS, Fyfe KL, Odoi A, Athukoralage A, Yiallourou SR, Wong FY. Dummy/pacifier use in preterm infants increases blood pressure and improves heart rate control. Pediatr Res. 2016;79(2):325–32.

194. Cohen M, Brown DR, Myers MM. Cardiovascular responses to pacifier experience and feeding in newborn infants. Dev Psychobiol. 2001;39:34–9.

195. Franco P, Scaillet S, Wermenbol V, Valente F, Groswasser J, Kahn A. The influence of a pacifier on infants' arousals from sleep. J Pediatr. 2000;136:775–9.

196. Hanzer M, Zotter H, Sauseng W, Pichler G, Pfurtscheller K, Mueller W, et al. Pacifier use does not alter the frequency or duration of spontaneous arousals in sleeping infants. Sleep Med. 2009;10:464–70.

197. Odoi A, Andrew S, Wong FY, Yiallourou SR, Horne RS. Pacifier use does not alter sleep and spontaneous arousal patterns in healthy term-born infants. Acta Paediatr. 2014;103(12): 1244–50.

198. Tonkin SL, Lui D, McIntosh CG, Rowley S, Knight DB, Gunn AJ. Effect of pacifier use on mandibular position in preterm infants. Acta Paediatr. 2007;96(10):1433–6.

199. Cozzi F, Albani R, Cardi E. A common pathophysiology for sudden cot death and sleep apnoea. "The vacuum-glossoptosis syndrome". Med Hypotheses. 1979;5(3):329–38.

200. Stratton K, Almario DA, Wizemann TM, McCormick MC. Immunization safety review: vaccinations and sudden unexpected death in infancy. Washington, DC: National Academies Press; 2003.

201. Mitchell EA, Stewart AW, Clements M. Immunisation and the sudden infant death syndrome. New Zealand Cot Death Study Group. Arch Dis Child. 1995;73(6):498–501.

202. Jonville-Bera AP, Autret-Leca E, Barbeillon F, Paris-Llado J. Sudden unexpected death in infants under 3 months of age and vaccination status- a case-control study. Br J Clin Pharmacol. 2001;51(3):271–6.

203. Fleming PJ, Blair PS, Platt MW, Tripp J, Smith IJ, Golding J. The UK accelerated immunisation programme and sudden unexpected death in infancy: case-control study. BMJ. 2001;322(7290):822.

204. Vennemann MM, Butterfass-Bahloul T, Jorch G, Brinkmann B, Findeisen M, Sauerland C, et al. Sudden infant death syndrome: no increased risk after immunisation. Vaccine. 2007;25(2):336–40.

205. Vennemann MM, Hoffgen M, Bajanowski T, Hense HW, Mitchell EA. Do immunisations reduce the risk for SIDS? A meta-analysis. Vaccine. 2007;25(26):4875–9.

206. Loy CS, Horne RS, Read PA, Cranage SM, Chau B, Adamson TM. Immunization has no effect on arousal from sleep in the newborn infant. J Paediatr Child Health. 1998;34(4):349–54.

Chapter 3
Safe Sleep Recommendations

Trina C. Salm Ward

Abbreviations

AAP   American Academy of Pediatrics
CDC   Centers for Disease Control and Prevention
CPSC Consumer Product Safety Commission
OR   Odds ratio
SIDS   Sudden infant death syndrome
SUID   Sudden unexpected infant death

Introduction

Each year in the United States, approximately 3600 infants die from sleep-related infant deaths (such as sudden infant death syndrome [SIDS], accidental suffocation and strangulation in bed, and ill-defined deaths) [1]. Parents can engage in behaviors to reduce the risk of these deaths [2]. Despite aggressive public education campaigns [3], the prevalence of risky sleep practices remains high, and there has been no decrease in rates of sleep-related infant deaths since 1999 [4, 5]. Research suggests that parents are more likely to adhere

T. C. Salm Ward (✉)
Department of Social Work, Helen Bader School of Social Welfare, University of Wisconsin-Milwaukee, Milwaukee, WI, USA
e-mail: salmward@uwm.edu

© Springer Nature Switzerland AG 2020   49
R. Y. Moon (ed.), *Infant Safe Sleep*,
https://doi.org/10.1007/978-3-030-47542-0_3

to recommendations for safe infant sleep made by their health-care providers [2, 6–10]. Thus, a primary focus for reducing rates of sleep-related infant deaths is health-care providers providing up-to-date, evidence-based recommendations for a safe infant sleeping environment [2].

Background

In the early 1990s, the American Academy of Pediatrics (AAP), a professional membership organization dedicated to the health of infants, created a Task Force on SIDS to review the emerging evidence for supine sleep position as a strategy to reduce the rate of SIDS [5].

For the past four decades, the Task Force has systematically reviewed the epidemiologic evidence on risk factors for SIDS and sleep-related suffocation, asphyxia, and entrapment among infants [5]. Based on this evidence, the Task Force drafts policy statements on recommendations for a safe infant sleeping environment, which are then vetted and approved by other AAP committees and sections and submitted to the AAP Executive Committee for final approval before publication [2]. Approximately every 5 years, the Task Force reviews the recent evidence and revises the policy statements as needed [2].

Prior to the 1990s, parents were routinely advised to place infants prone for sleep [11]. The original 1992 policy statement recommended the back sleeping position [12], and the subsequent "Back to Sleep" campaign (now known as Safe to Sleep®) by the National Institute of Health and Human Development [3] was associated with a steady increase in the use of the back sleep positon and a concomitant dramatic decline in rates of sleep-related infant deaths [2]. As more epidemiologic studies were published, subsequent policy statements expanded recommendations to include other factors such as sleep surface and sleep environment [2, 13–16].

The current (2016) version synthesizes evidence from 400 research articles into a 12-page policy statement outlining the recommendations for a safe infant sleeping environment [2]. An accompanying technical report provides a more detailed discussion of the evidence [5]. Recommendations are based on epidemiologic studies that include infants up to 1 year of age; therefore, recommendations are for the first year after birth, unless otherwise specified [2]. Evidence for each recommendation was assessed based on the Strength-of-Recommendation Taxonomy [17]. A-level recommendations are based on good-quality patient-oriented evidence, B-level recommendations mean there is inconsistent or limited-quality patient-oriented evidence, and C-level recommendations mean they are based on consensus, expert opinion, disease-oriented evidence, usual practice, or case series for studies of diagnosis, treatment, prevention, or screening [2]. Patient-oriented evidence measures outcomes that matter to patients, such as morbidity, mortality, symptom improvement, cost reduction, and quality of life [2, 17]. The recommendations are summarized below, along with a summary of the evidence supporting each recommendation. Recommendations are briefly summarized in Table 3.1.

TABLE 3.1 Summary of recommendations for a safe infant sleep environment

A-level recommendations

1. Place infant back (supine) to sleep every time baby sleeps.

2. Use a flat, firm sleep surface.

3. Breastfeeding reduces risk of SIDS.

4. Infants should sleep in the parents' room on a separate sleep surface.

5. Keep soft objects and loose bedding away from infant's sleep area.

6. Consider offering a pacifier during sleep.

7. Avoid smoke exposure during pregnancy and after birth.

(continued)

TABLE 3.1 (continued)

8. Avoid alcohol and illicit drug use during pregnancy and after birth.

9. Avoid overheating and head covering.

10. Pregnant women should receive regular prenatal care.

11. Infants should be immunized in accordance with AAP and CDC recommendations.

12. Do not use heart or breathing monitors in the home as a strategy to reduce SIDS risk.

13. Providers should endorse and model SIDS risk-reduction recommendations.

14. Media and manufacturers should follow safe sleep guidelines in messaging and advertising.

15. Pediatricians and primary care providers should actively participate in the safe to sleep® campaign.

B-level recommendations

16. Avoid products that go against safe sleep recommendations, especially those that claim to prevent or reduce the risk of SIDS.

17. Give baby supervised, awake tummy time to facilitate development.

C-level recommendations

18. Continue research and surveillance on the mechanisms of sleep-related infant deaths.

19. There is no evidence to recommend swaddling to reduce SIDS risk.

Adapted from American Academy of Pediatrics Task Force on Sudden Infant Death Syndrome [2]

Recommendations to Reduce the Risk of SIDS and Other Sleep-Related Infant Deaths

A-Level Recommendations

A-level recommendations are based on good-quality patient-oriented evidence [2].

1. *Back to sleep every time baby sleeps.* (For additional details, please see Chap. 5.)

Infants should be placed supine for sleep (wholly on the back) for every sleep until 1 year of age [2]. Prone or side sleep position increases risk for hypercapnia, hypoxia, and overheating and alters the autonomic control of the infant cardiovascular system which may result in decreased cerebral oxygenation (see Chap. 2). The side position is just as risky as the prone position due to the probability of an infant more easily rolling to the prone position; epidemiological evidence has demonstrated that the odds ratio (OR) for SIDS associated with prone position ranges from 2.3 to 13.1, and one US study found SIDS risk associated with the side (OR 2.0) and prone (OR 2.6) position to be statistically similar [5]. Moreover, the risk of prone placement for infants who are not accustomed to that position is higher than the risk for those usually placed prone (adjusted OR: 8.7–45.4) [5]. A 2017 editorial further summarizes recent evidence on the mechanisms of prone sleep that increase risk of infant death [18].

Preterm infants should also be placed supine as soon as clinical status has stabilized and well before the infant will be discharged home [5] so the infant becomes acclimated to supine sleeping before discharge and to model supine sleep for parents [2].

2. *Use a flat, firm sleep surface.* (For additional details, please see Chap. 8.)

Infants should be placed on a firm sleep surface (such as a crib mattress) covered by a fitted sheet with no other bedding or soft objects [2]. The Task Force defines "firm" as a surface that does not indent or conform to the shape of the infant's head when the infant is laid on the surface [2]. Soft mattresses, including memory foam mattresses, can indent or conform to the infant's body which could increase the chance of infant rebreathing or suffocation. It is recommended that infants sleep in a crib, bassinet, portable crib, or play yard that meets the safety standards of the Consumer Product Safety Commission (CPSC, cpsc.gov).

Pillows, cushions, mattress toppers, sheep skins, quilts, or comforters should not be used because of increased risk of suffocation [2]. Infants should not be placed for sleep on beds, nor should they be placed for sleep on even fully inflated air mattresses, because of the risk of entrapment and suffocation [2, 19].

Infant sleep surfaces should be flat (horizontally placed). In 2019, the CPSC recalled several models of inclined sleepers due to infant deaths [20]. Recently, the CPSC proposed a rule for infant sleep products that would ban any incline above 10 degrees, based on a biomechanics study that found infants in inclined sleep products were at higher risk of suffocation in these products compared to a flat crib mattress [21]. Similarly, sitting devices, such as car seats, strollers, swings, infant carriers, and infant slings, should not be used for routine sleep. If an infant falls asleep during travel, they should ideally be moved to a flat, firm surface as soon as possible after travel is concluded [22]. Younger infants (i.e., those younger than 4 months) are particularly at risk in inclined sleepers and sitting devices.

Parents may consider other products for infant sleep. Bedside sleepers are attached to the side of the parental bed; the CPSC has published safety standards for these products [23]. In-bed sleepers, used in the parental bed, are also easily available, but there are currently no CPSC safety standards for these. A recent *Consumer Reports* investigation found that at least 12 infant deaths between 2012 and 2018 were associated with in-bed sleepers [24].

3. *Breastfeeding is recommended.* (For additional details, please see Chap. 7).

Feeding breastmilk to an infant (via direct breastfeeding or providing expressed milk) for at least 2 months is associated with a reduced risk of SIDS [25]. Breastfeeding does not need to be exclusive to confer this protective effect. Breastmilk reduces the risk of SIDS in multiple ways – breastfed infants are more easily aroused from sleep and have a lower incidence of diarrhea and other infections associated with increased vulnerability to SIDS, and breastfeeding results in a gut microbiome that supports a normally functioning immune system [5]. Mothers are thus encouraged to breastfeed as much and as long as possible.

4. *Infants should sleep in the parents' room, close to the parents' bed, but on a separate surface designed for infants, ideally for the first year of life but at least for the first 6 months.* (For additional details, please see Chap. 6).

Current evidence suggests that sleeping in the parents' room on a separate surface is safer than either bed-sharing or having the infant sleep in a separate room [5]. Because rates of sleep-related infant deaths, particularly those that occur during bed-sharing, are highest in the first 6 months of life, room-sharing without bed-sharing is recommended for at least the first 6 months. Placing the infant's sleep surface adjacent to the parents' bed will allow easy access to feed and monitor the infant [2].

Two recent systematic reviews have suggested differences between infants who bed-share and those who do not bed-share. The first systematic review of physiological studies on bed-sharing found that bed-sharing infants had increased arousals, warmer temperatures, and longer breastfeeding duration [26]. The second systematic review of the evidence related to sleep-related infant deaths suggests that the lethal mechanisms for bed-sharing infants may be different than the lethal mechanisms for infants sleeping alone [27].

There are specific bed-sharing circumstances that *substantially increase risk* of infant death or injury [2]:

- When an adult bed-sharer is a current smoker or if the mother smoked during pregnancy.
- When the infant is younger than 4 months (regardless of whether parent is smoker or not).
- When the infant was born preterm and/or low birth weight (regardless of whether parent is smoker or not).
- When an adult bed-sharer has used sedating medicines (e.g., pain medicines), alcohol, or illicit drugs.
- When an adult bed-sharer may have difficulty with arousal because of fatigue.
- On a sofa, couch, or armchair.
- On any other soft surface, including but not limited to waterbed, old mattress, or air mattress.
- When soft bedding accessories, such as pillows or blankets, are present.
- When those bed-sharing with the infant are not the infant's parents.

The adult bed is a safer place to feed an infant than a sofa, couch, or armchair. Parents are encouraged to bring the infant into the bed to feed and then move the infant back to a separate sleep surface when the parent is ready to fall asleep. If the parent should fall asleep while feeding, the infant should be moved to a separate sleep surface as soon as the parent awakens.

If there is concern that a parent may fall asleep in bed while feeding the infant, parents should proactively prepare the bed to minimize risk to the infant [2]:

- Remove pillows, loose sheets, blankets, or any other items that could obstruct infant breathing or cause overheating.
- Follow other safe sleep recommendations outlined in this chapter (e.g., supine sleep position).
- As soon as parent awakens, she should place infant back on a separate sleep surface.

5. *Keep soft objects and loose bedding away from the infant's sleep area.* (For additional details, please see Chap. 8.)

Soft objects include items such as pillows, stuffed toys, quilts, comforters, blankets, nonfitted sheets, sheepskins, bumper pads, and towels, all of which can obstruct an infant's nose and mouth and increase risk of SIDS, suffocation, or entrapment [2]. Bedding increases the risk of SIDS five-fold; when the infant is sleeping prone, this risk increases to 21-fold [5]. Soft and loose bedding can also increase the risk of accidental suffocation. A recent analysis from the Centers for Disease Control and Prevention (CDC)s Sudden Unexpected Infant Death (SUID) Case Registry found that 69% of suffocation deaths were attributed to soft bedding [28]. Soft bedding-related suffocation deaths occurred most often in a prone position (82%), in an adult bed (49%), and with a blanket (or blankets) obstructing the airway (34%) [28].

Infant sleep clothing, in layers if needed to keep the infant warm, is preferable to blankets and other coverings, as this can decrease the risk of head covering or entrapment with a blanket [2].

6. *Consider offering a pacifier at naptime and bedtime.*

Pacifiers have a protective effect on the incidence of SIDS, although the mechanism is not yet clear [2]. Several studies have found the effect is particularly (50–90%) protective when a pacifier is used at the time of the last sleep period [5]. This protective effect continues even if the pacifier falls out of the infant's mouth; thus, it does not need to be reinserted once the infant falls asleep [2].

Pacifiers should not be hung around an infant's neck and should not be attached to stuffed toys or other items to avoid risk of strangulation, suffocation, and choking risk [2].

For breastfeeding infants, pacifiers should not be introduced until breastfeeding is firmly established [2]. A recent Cochrane review comparing pacifier use and nonuse in healthy term breastfeeding infants found that pacifier use did not impact partial or exclusive breastfeeding rates at 3 and 4 months [5].

7. Avoid smoke exposure during pregnancy and after birth.

Smoke exposure, both in utero and after birth, increases SIDS risk. The independent contribution of prenatal and postnatal smoke exposure is difficult to separate, as most mothers who smoke also smoked during pregnancy [2]. A recent analysis of the CDC Linked Birth/Infant Death data set suggested that 22% of SUIDs in the United States could be attributed to maternal smoking during pregnancy and that risk of SUID increased with each additional cigarette smoked per day [29]. Cochrane reviews summarize the current evidence regarding smoking cessation interventions in pregnancy [30,31]. A recent prospective, multicenter, observational study found a significantly higher risk for SIDS among infants who were prenatally exposed to both alcohol and cigarettes beyond the first trimester (relative risk [RR]: 11.79) compared to infants who were unexposed, exposed to alcohol (RR: 3.95) or cigarettes (RR: 4.86) alone, or when mother reported quitting early in pregnancy [32]. Thus, providers should continue to encourage women to stop smoking and alcohol use throughout the pregnancy.

8. *Avoid alcohol and illicit drug use during pregnancy and after birth.*

Multiple studies have found maternal alcohol use and binge drinking are associated with increased risk of SIDS [2]. As noted in #7 above, the combination of prenatal alcohol and cigarette exposure also significantly increases risk for SIDS [32]. Other studies have found increased risk of SIDS with the use of illicit drugs, such as cannabis, opiates such as methadone and heroin, and cocaine [5]. Cochrane reviews summarize the current evidence regarding drug and alcohol treatment during pregnancy [33–35].

9. *Avoid overheating and head covering.*

In general, infants should have no more than one layer of additional clothing beyond what an adult would wear to be comfortable [2]. Studies have demonstrated an increased risk of SIDS with overheating; due to varying definitions of overheating in epidemiologic studies, it is difficult to provide specific room temperature guidelines [2]. Parents and care-givers should avoid covering the infant's face and head during sleep [2].

10. *Pregnant women should seek and receive regular prenatal care.*

Substantial epidemiologic evidence has linked receipt of regular prenatal care to a lower risk of SIDS [2]. Pregnant women should receive prenatal care visits as outlined in the joint AAP and American College of Obstetricians and Gynecologists guidelines [2, 36].

11. *Infants should be immunized in accordance with AAP and CDC recommendations.*

There is no evidence of a causal relationship between immunizations and SIDS [2]. Appropriately immunized infants are at lower risk for SIDS (see Chap. 2).

12. *Do not use heart or breathing monitors in the home as a strategy to reduce the risk of SIDS.*

There are no data that use of home cardiorespiratory monitors or other commercial devices designed to monitor infant vital signs reduces the risk of SIDS [5]. While devices may be prescribed for use at home or used in hospital, they have not been shown to detect infants at risk of SIDS [2]. Anecdotal evidence suggests that some parents may mistakenly believe that using a home monitor will protect their infant from risk of unexpected death and thus may believe it is acceptable to place their infant prone [18].

13. *Providers should endorse and model the SIDS risk-reduction recommendations from birth.*

Health-care professionals should model and implement all risk-reduction recommendations; for hospitalized infants, these recommendations should be implemented as soon as an infant is medically stable to allow adequate time for the infant and parents to become accustomed to a safe sleep environment well before anticipated hospital discharge [2]. All providers should receive ongoing training on safe infant sleep and provide anticipatory guidance regarding safe sleep at well-child visits throughout infancy [2]. Hospitals and child care agencies should ensure that written policies are consistent with the most recent safe sleep guidelines and that infant bassinets and cribs meet all current safety standards [2].

14. *Media and manufacturers should follow safe sleep guidelines in their messaging and advertising.*

The Internet and social media have become primary and trusted sources of information for parents when making infant sleep decisions [2, 10]. However, media and advertising messages that do not comply with safe sleep recommendations can cause confusion for parents [2].

15. *Continue the Safe to Sleep® campaign, focusing on ways to reduce risk of sleep-related infant deaths. Pediatricians and other primary care providers should actively participate in this campaign.*

B-Level Recommendations

B-level recommendations are those that have inconsistent or limited-quality patient-oriented evidence [2].

16. *Avoid products that go against safe sleep recommendations, especially those that claim to prevent or reduce the risk of SIDS.* (For additional details, please see Chap. 9.)

While some devices claim to reduce SIDS (e.g., wedges and positioners or devices to be used in the adult bed), there is no evidence that any of them reduce the risk of SIDS [2]. Safe sleep practices should be followed with the use of any products.

17. *Give baby supervised, awake tummy time to facilitate development and to minimize development of positional plagiocephaly.*

Prone positioning, or tummy time, while the infant is awake and observed, is recommended to help prevent positional pla-giocephaly by the AAP Committee on Practice and Ambulatory Medicine and Section on Neurologic Surgery and the Task Force on SIDS [2].

C-Level Recommendations

C-level recommendations are based on consensus, expert opinion, disease-oriented evidence, usual practice, or case series for studies of diagnosis, treatment, prevention, or screening [2].

18. *Continue research and surveillance on the risk factors, causes, and pathophysiologic mechanisms of SIDS and other sleep-related infant deaths, with the ultimate goal of eliminating those deaths entirely.*

Research has contributed to a better, yet still limited, understanding of the etiology and pathophysiological basis of sleep-related infant deaths. Ongoing surveillance of these deaths, for example, the CDC SUID Case Registry, can help elucidate mechanisms of these deaths [37]. Recently, the international infant death research community conducted an international consensus project among 25 countries to iden-tify priority research areas [38]. Further, education campaigns and innovative interventions need to be rigorously evaluated [7, 8]. These efforts require funding by federal and private funding agencies.

19. *There is no evidence to recommend swaddling as a strategy to reduce the risk of SIDS.*

Swaddling (i.e., wrapping the infant in a light blanket) is a frequent practice for calming an infant. It may allow an infant to more easily sleep supine. However, infants are at much greater risk of death if they are swaddled and placed in or roll into the prone position [2]. Swaddled infants should always be placed on their back, and when an infant begins to attempt to roll (whether swaddled or unswaddled), swaddling should be discontinued [2]. A recent meta-analysis of SIDS risk for swaddled infants reinforced the advice to avoid prone or side positions for sleep and suggested that the risk of death increased with age, peaking for infants aged 6 months or older [39].

References

1. Centers for Disease Control and Prevention: About SUID and SIDS. 2018. https://www.cdc.gov/sids/about/. Accessed 01 Oct 2019.
2. American Academy of Pediatrics Task Force on Sudden Infant Death Syndrome. SIDS and other sleep-related deaths: Updated 2016 recommendations for a safe infant sleeping environment. Pediatrics. 2016;138(5):e20162938. https://doi.org/10.1542/peds.2016-2938.
3. National Institute of Child Health and Human Development: Safe to sleep education campaign. 2019. http://safetosleep.nichd.nih.gov/. Accessed 01 Oct 2019.
4. Bombard JM, Kortsmit K, Warner L, Shapiro-Mendoza CK, Cox S, Kroelinger CD, et al. Trends and disparities in infant safe sleep practices – United States, 2009–2015. Morb Mortal Wkly Rep. 2018;67(1):39–46. https://doi.org/10.15585/mmwr.mm6701e1.
5. Moon RY, American Academy of Pediatrics Task Force on Sudden Infant Death Syndrome. SIDS and other sleep-related infant deaths: Evidence base for 2016 updated recommendations for a safe infant sleeping environment. Pediatrics. 2016;138(5):e20162940. https://doi.org/10.1542/peds.2016-2940.
6. Hwang SS, Rybin DV, Heeren TC, Colson ER, Corwin MJ. Trust in sources of advice about infant care practices: the SAFE study. Matern Child Health J. 2016;20(9):1956–64. https://doi.org/10.1007/s10995-016-2011-3.
7. Moon RY, Hauck FR, Colson ER. Safe infant sleep interventions: what is the evidence for successful behavior change? Curr Pediatr Rev. 2016;12(1):67–75. https://doi.org/10.2174/1573396311666151026110148.
8. Salm Ward TC, Balfour G. Infant safe sleep interventions, 1990–2015: a review. J Comm Health. 2016;41(1):180–96. https://doi.org/10.1007/s10900-015-0060-y.

9. Walcott RL, Salm Ward TC, Ingels JB, Llewellyn NA, Miller TJ, Corso PS. A statewide hospital-based safe infant sleep initiative: measurement of parental knowledge and behavior. J Comm Health. 2018;43(3):534–42. https://doi.org/10.1007/s10900-017-0449-x.

10. Moon, RY, Mathews A, Oden R, Carlin R. A qualitative analysis of how mothers' social networks are established and used to make infant care decisions. Clin Pediatr. 2019;58(9):985–92. https://doi.org/10.1177/0009922819845332.

11. Gilbert R, Salanti G, Harden M, See S. Infant sleeping position and the sudden infant death syndrome: systematic review of observational studies and historical review of recommendations from 1940 to 2002. Int J Epidemiol. 2005;34(4):874–87. https://doi.org/10.1093/ije/dyi088.

12. American Academy of Pediatrics. Positioning and SIDS. Pediatrics. 1992;39:1120–6.

13. American Academy of Pediatrics. Does bed sharing affect the risk of SIDS? Pediatrics. 1997;100(2):272. https://doi.org/10.1542/peds.100.2.272.

14. American Academy of Pediatrics. Changing concepts of sudden infant death syndrome: implications for infant sleeping environment and sleep position. Pediatrics. 2000;105(3):650–6. https://doi.org/10.1542/peds.105.3.650.

15. American Academy of Pediatrics. The changing concept of sudden infant death syndrome (SIDS): diagnostic coding shifts, controversies regarding the sleeping environment, and new variables to consider in reducing risk. Pediatrics. 2005;116(5):1245–55. https://doi.org/10.1542/peds.2005-1499.

16. American Academy of Pediatrics Task Force on Sudden Infant Death Syndrome. SIDS and other sleep-related infant deaths: expansion of recommendations for a safe infant sleeping environment. Pediatrics. 2011;128(5):1030–9. https://doi.org/10.1542/peds.2011-2284.

17. Ebell MH, Siwek J, Weiss BD, Woolf SH, Susman J, Ewigman B, et al. Strength of recommendation taxonomy (SORT): a patient-centered approach to grading evidence in the medical literature. Am Fam Physician. 2004;69(3):548–56. https://www.aafp.org/afp/2004/0201/p548.html.

18. Fleming P, Blair P, Pease A. Why or how does the prone sleep position increase the risk of unexpected and unexplained infant death? Arch Dis Child Fetal Neonatal Ed. 2017;102(6):F472–3. https://doi.org/10.1136/archdischild-2017-313331.

19. Doering JJ, Salm Ward TC. The interface among poverty, air mattress industry trends, policy, and infant safety. Am J Public Health. 2017;107(6):945–9. https://doi.org/10.2105/AJPH.2017.303709.

20. U.S. Consumer Product Safety Commission: Safe sleep - cribs and infant infant products information center. 2019. https://www.cpsc.gov/safesleep. Accessed 01 Oct 2019.

21. Frankel TC. Study concludes design of Rock n' Play, other infant sleepers led to deaths. 2019. https://www.washingtonpost.com/business/2019/10/17/study-concludes-design-rock-n-play-other-infant-sleepers-led-deaths/. Accessed 25 Oct 2019.

22. Liaw P, Moon RY, Han A, Colvin JD. Infant deaths in sitting devices. Pediatrics. 2019;143(6):320182576. https://doi.org/10.1542/peds.2018-2576.

23. U.S. Consumer Product Safety Commission: Safety standard for beside sleepers. 2014. https://www.cpsc.gov/Regulations-Laws%2D%2DStandards/Rulemaking/Final-and-Proposed-Rules/Bedside-Sleepers. Accessed 01 Oct 2019.

24. Peachman RR. More infant sleep products linked to deaths, a Consumer Reports investigation finds. 2019. https://www.consumerreports.org/child-safety/more-infant-sleep-products-linked-to-deaths/. Accessed 25 Oct 2019.

25. Thompson JMD, Tanabe K, Moon RY, Mitchell EA, McGarvey C, Tappin D, Blair PS, Hauck FR. Duration of breastfeeding and risk of SIDS: an individual participant data meta-analysis. Pediatrics. 2017;140(5):e20171324. https://doi.org/10.1542/peds.2017-1324.

26. Baddock SA, Purnell MT, Blair PS, Pease AS, Edler DE, Galland BC. The influence of bedsharing on infant physiology, breastfeeding and behavior: a systematic review. Sleep Med Rev. 2019;43:106–17. https://doi.org/10.1016/j.smrv.2018.10.007.

27. Collins-Praino LE, Byard RW. Infants who die in shared sleeping situations differ from those who die while sleeping alone. Acta Pediatrica. 2019;108:611–4. https://doi.org/10.1111/apa.14692.

28. Erck Lambert AB, Parks SE, Cottengim C, Faulkner M, Hauck FR, Shapiro-Mendoza CK. Sleep-related infant suffocation deaths attributable to soft bedding, overlay, and wedging. Pediatrics. 2019;143(5):e20183408. https://doi.org/10.1542/peds.2018-3408.

29. Anderson TM, Lavista Ferres JM, Ren SY, Moon RY, Goldstein RD, Ramirez JM, et al. Maternal smoking before and dur-

ing pregnancy and the risk of Sudden Unexpected Infant Death. Pediatrics. 2019;143(4):e20183325. https://doi.org/10.1542/peds.2018-3325.

30. Chamberlain C, O'Mara-Eves A, Porter J, Coleman T, Perlen SM, Thomas J, et al. Psychosocial interventions for supporting women to stop smoking in pregnancy. Cochrane Database Syst Rev. 2017;2. https://doi.org/10.1002/14651858.CD001055.pub5.

31. Coleman T, Chamberlain C, Davey MA, Cooper SE, Leonardi-Bee J. Pharmacological interventions for promoting smoking cessation during pregnancy. Cochrane Database Syst Rev. 2015;12 https://doi.org/10.1002/14651858.CD010078.pub2.

32. Elliott AJ, Kinney HC, Haynes RL, Dempers JD, Wright C, Fifer WP, et al. Concurrent prenatal drinking and smoking increases risk for SIDS: safe passage study report. EClinicalMedicine. 2020;100247. https://doi.org/10.1016/j.eclinm.2019.100247.

33. Minozzi S, Amato L, Bellisario C, Ferri M, Davoli M. Maintenance agonist treatments for opiate-dependent pregnant women. Cochrane Database Syst Rev. 2013;12. https://doi.org/10.1002/14651858.CD006318.pub3.

34. Stade BC, Bailey C, Dzendoletas D, Sgro M, Dowswell T, Bennett D. Psychological and/or educational interventions for reducing alcohol consumption in pregnant women and women planning pregnancy. Cochrane Database Syst Rev. 2009;2. https://doi.org/10.1002/14651858.CD004228.pub2.

35. Terplan M, Ramanadhan S, Locke A, Longinaker N, Lui S. Psychosocial interventions for pregnant women in outpatient illicit drug treatment programs compared to other interventions. Cochrane Database Syst Rev. 2015;4. https://doi.org/10.1002/14651858.CD006037.pub3.

36. American Academy of Pediatrics Committee on Fetus and Newborn, American College of Obstetricians and Gynecologists Committee on Obstetric Practice. Guidelines for perinatal care, 8th ed. Elk Grove Village: American Academy of Pediatrics; 2017. https://ebooks.aappublications.org/content/guidelines-for-perinatal-care-8th-edition.

37. Shapiro-Mendoza CK, Camperlengo LT, Kim SY, Covington T. The sudden unexpected infant death case registry: a method to improve surveillance. Pediatrics. 2012;129(2):e486–93. https://doi.org/10.1542/peds.2011-0854.

38. Hauck FR, McEntire BL, Raven LK, Bates FL, Lyus LA, Willett AM, et al. Research priorities in sudden unexpected infant death:

an international consensus. Pediatrics. 2017;140(2):e20163514. https://doi.org/10.1542/peds.2016-3514.

39. Pease AS, Fleming PJ, Hauck FR, Moon RY, Horne RSC, L'Hoir MP, et al. Swaddling and the risk of sudden infant death syndrome: a meta-analysis. Pediatrics. 2016;137(6):e20153275. https://doi.org/10.1542/peds.2015-3275.

Chapter 4
Parent Decision-Making and How to Influence Decisions

Trina C. Salm Ward and Rachel Y. Moon

Introduction

Parents make multiple decisions on a daily basis, and healthcare providers may not fully understand the reasons behind specific decisions. We know that despite knowledge of safe sleep recommendations, families may adjust their practices, even if they know that these practices are inconsistent with the recommendations, to meet their unique needs [1–14]. We also know that what parents intend to do before the baby is born may change after the baby is brought home [15–18] and that some families who make decisions inconsistent with recommendations may feel stigmatized about their decision-making and thus may be reluctant to discuss their infant sleep practices with providers [11, 19–21].

Before one has a conversation with a parent, it may be helpful to understand a little bit about how the parent made

T. C. Salm Ward
Department of Social Work, Helen Bader School of Social Welfare, University of Wisconsin-Milwaukee, Milwaukee, WI, USA
e-mail: salmward@uwm.edu

R. Y. Moon (✉)
Department of Pediatrics, University of Virginia School of Medicine, Charlottesville, VA, USA
e-mail: rym4z@virginia.edu

© Springer Nature Switzerland AG 2020   67
R. Y. Moon (ed.), *Infant Safe Sleep*,
https://doi.org/10.1007/978-3-030-47542-0_4

a specific decision. In this chapter, we describe some theoretical frameworks that may help explain how parents make decisions about infant sleep practices and include examples from the perspective of current infant sleep practice research. We propose a decision-making flowchart that incorporates this information and discuss ways to influence parental decision-making within the context of this decision-making flowchart.

Theoretical Perspectives

Socio-ecological Model

The socio-ecological model is a useful framework to understand the levels of influence on infant sleep decisions [10, 22, 23]. This model posits that families' infant sleep practices influence and are influenced by factors at the infant, maternal, family and household, and community/societal levels (Fig. 4.1) [10]. The National Action Partnership to Promote Safe Sleep (NAPPSS) also uses the socio-ecological model in its conceptual model to help make safe sleep a national norm (http://www.nappss.org).

FIGURE 4.1 Socio-ecological model applied to infant sleep practices. (Modified from Ref. [10]. The socio-ecological model suggests that we should think about how each of these levels might affect a parent's decision. For example, if the home does not have adequate heat or the parent is worried about neighborhood safety, she may choose to bring the baby into her bed. In this example, just giving the advice "the American Academy of Pediatrics recommends that babies sleep on a separate surface" will not address the concerns that lead to her decision to bed-share. This model reinforces the importance of asking families about their perceptions and reasons behind infant sleep practices. The socio-ecological model also suggests that to address complex health behaviors such as infant sleep practices, comprehensive multilevel approaches must be considered [10, 23]

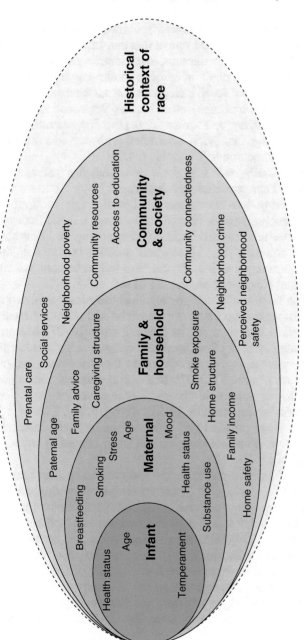

The *infant level* includes infant characteristics such as age, health status, and temperament that may influence (or be influenced by) a parent's decision. For example, parents may bed-share to monitor an ill infant or to soothe a crying infant [11].

The *maternal level* includes maternal characteristics, for example, maternal age, breastfeeding, stress, and mood (e.g., depressive symptoms or anxiety) [10]. For example, young maternal age has been associated with use of non-supine sleep position and soft bedding [24, 25].

The *family and household level* includes paternal and familial characteristics and household factors. For example, bed-sharing has been associated with single motherhood, experiencing partner-related stress, moving more than once since the infant's birth, household crowding, and household safety concerns [10, 11]. Mothers' social networks (i.e., their trusted family and friends) can also influence practices such as infant sleep position and use of soft bedding [26].

The *community and society level* includes neighborhood conditions and access to opportunities and resources, such as education, employment, and health care [10, 27]. Maternal education, income level, and health care are included in this level because they serve as a proxy for other variables, such as issues of access [10, 27]. Bed-sharing has been associated with lower household income, lower education levels, and concerns about neighborhood safety [10, 11]. Use of non-supine sleep position and soft bedding has been associated with lower household income and lower education levels [10, 17, 24, 25].

The *historical context of race*, suggested by Alio and colleagues [28], is helpful in understanding racial disparities in infant sleep practices and incorporates the impact that personally mediated and structural racism has had on Black Americans [10]. Historical experiences of racism (e.g., Tuskegee Syphilis study [29]), which can be connected to historical trauma, can affect the level of trust that infant caregivers place in advice from health-care providers or other professions that have a history of oppressing minority groups, in particular, Black Americans. The Institute of Medicine's

2003 report, *Unequal Treatment*, found racial disparities in both health outcomes and quality of health care and that racism, defined as a social construct that refers to institutional and individual practices that create and reinforce oppressive systems [30, 31], is a contributor to these disparities [32]. Studies have documented that Black Americans may still mistrust US health-care providers and systems [33–36]. Others have found higher levels of adherence to safe sleep recommendations if they are reinforced by health-care providers [13, 37–39].

The Integrated Behavioral Model

The integrated behavioral model (IBM) is a model of behavior that synthesizes multiple health behavior models, including the theory of planned behavior, theory of reasoned action, social cognitive theory, and the health belief model [40, 41]. The IBM suggests that when thinking about actually performing a behavior (e.g., placing the baby supine), intentions remain the most important determinant of behavior. Intention to perform the behavior is influenced by attitudes, perceived norms, and personal agency. However, additional factors that also influence whether or not a parent performs the behavior include knowledge and skills, salience of the behavior, environmental constraints, and habit (Fig. 4.2).

Below, we briefly summarize the main components of the integrated behavioral model and how they apply to decision-making about infant sleep practices.

Intention refers to a person's readiness to engage in a behavior, or the person's estimate of their likelihood of actually performing the behavior [41]. Intention can be viewed as a continuum from a strong intention *not* to perform a behavior to a strong intention *to* perform a behavior [42]. A parent may thus state, "I will place my baby on her back to sleep," or "I plan to place my baby in his crib."

Attitude refers to the person's overall agreeableness toward performing the behavior and includes two constructs: experi-

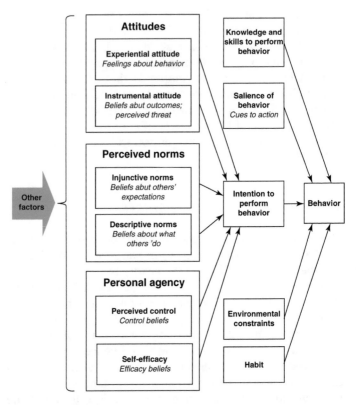

FIGURE 4.2 The integrated behavioral model. (Reprinted with permission from Ref. [40])

ential attitude and instrumental attitude [40]. *Experiential attitude* refers to a person's feelings about a behavior, i.e., their emotional or "gut" reaction to the thought of performing the behavior [42]. If a person has a positive emotional reaction to the thought of performing the behavior, he or she is more likely to perform the behavior than if there is a negative emotional reaction to the thought of performing the behavior [40]. For example, mothers may make decisions about infant sleep based on their "maternal instinct," or what they feel is right, or best, for their baby [11]. A feeling of "this feels right" or "this feels best for my baby" would be a positive feeling about a behavior, such as placing supine to sleep or on a separate sleep surface. Alternatively, if maternal instincts conflict with safe sleep recommendations, mothers may be less willing to engage in the behavior. One study found that mothers who had "positive attitudes about the prone sleep position (i.e., agreed with the statements that putting the infant in the prone position for sleep would be healthy for the infant, be pleasant for the infant, be good for the infant, make the infant safer, make the infant more comfortable, and/or keep the infant from choking) were much more likely to choose the prone position" [17]. *Instrumental attitude* refers to a person's behavioral beliefs or beliefs and expectations about the costs and benefits (perceived outcomes) of performing the behavior [40, 42]. For example, if a person believes that a particular behavior will lead to positive outcomes or that those positive outcomes/benefits outweigh the costs of performing the behavior, there will be a positive attitude toward the behavior [40]. However, if a person believes that the behavior will have negative outcomes or that the costs outweigh the benefits of performing the behavior, there will be a negative attitude toward the behavior. A parent who decides to place the baby prone may believe that the immediate benefits of the baby sleeping more soundly outweigh the long-term benefits of practicing safe sleep [42]. However, if a parent believes that placing the infant supine will reduce the risk of the infant dying and that this benefit outweighs the cost of placing the baby supine (e.g., the baby will not sleep as long), he or she is more likely to place the infant supine.

Perceived threat is a component of the health belief model and has particular relevance to infant sleep practices. Perceived threat includes two components, *perceived susceptibility* to the negative health outcome (in this case, infant death) and *perceived severity*, or seriousness of that outcome [43, 44]. Parents may perceive a low susceptibility of death, for example, because they feel their infant is immune to SIDS [39] or that the chances of the baby dying are very low [2, 45, 47]. Thus, a focus of safe sleep education is to help parents realize that every infant is potentially at risk of death [39]. Providers could describe susceptibility in clear terms, for example, "every week, three infants die of sleep-related causes in this state" [18], or communicate that the risk of sleep-related deaths is significantly higher than other leading causes of childhood deaths [42].

Perceived norms refer to the social pressure a person feels to perform (or not perform) a particular behavior and include two constructs: injunctive norms and descriptive norms [40]. *Injunctive norms* refer to a person's belief about others' expectations, or what other people think they should do, and a person's motivation to comply with those others' expectations – e.g., "everyone thinks that I should breast-feed" [47]. Thus, if the baby's grandmother tells a mother that she should place the baby to sleep on his stomach because he will sleep better, the mother may be motivated to comply with that advice because the grandmother has successfully raised several children and so the mother trusts her advice, because the mother relies on grandmother to assist in child care and other resources, and/or because the mother may feel negatively judged by the grandmother if she does not comply [9]. She would thus be complying with the injunctive norm. Parents receive advice and information about what they should do for infant sleep from multiple sources, including family, health-care providers, friends, and media [9, 13, 17, 38, 39, 48–53]. These trusted sources of information comprise the parent's social network and illustrate the extended influence of injunctive norms. While the health-care professional remains an important source of information, the influence of the social network is powerful and cannot be ignored. Mothers get a clear sense of what practices are prevalent ("normal") and acceptable – i.e., what the social norms are – from those around them, and they are more likely to adhere to these social norms, even if these are discordant with health-care recommendations.

Descriptive norms refer to a person's beliefs about others' behaviors, or what others are doing – e.g., "everyone else is breastfeeding" [47]. If a mother sees bumper pads being sold in baby stores and advertised in parenting magazines and because she sees popular magazine photos of celebrity nurseries with bumper pads in the crib, she may conclude that this is "the thing to do" for one's baby and purchase the bumper pads to place in her infant's crib. She is complying with the descriptive norm.

Another example of perceived norms is that new parents are commonly asked, "Is your baby sleeping through the night yet?" This leads to a parental expectation that the infant *should* be sleeping through the night and the perception that their infant is somehow lacking if there are still night wakings. Particularly because many parents do not realize that a normal infant needs frequent night wakings for frequent feedings (partly because of the small size of an infant's stomach) [54–56], this perception may lead to a parent changing an infant's sleep position to prone so that the infant will "sleep better."

Personal agency is a person's own influence on their behavior and includes two constructs: perceived behavioral control and self-efficacy [57]. *Perceived behavioral control*, or control beliefs, refers to the extent to which a person believes that he or she is capable of or has control over performing the behavior [47]. *Self-efficacy*, or efficacy beliefs, is defined as confidence in one's own ability to take action and belief that one's actions can make a difference in the outcomes [58]. Parents who live in dangerous neighborhoods or vermin-infested apartments may not feel they have control over the safety of the neighborhood or home and may bed-share in an effort to protect their infant from these dangers. Other parents may not feel they have control over infant temperament and may place the baby prone because it makes the baby happy. Parents may believe that SIDS occurs randomly or is "God's will" and thus have a lower degree of self-efficacy regarding their ability to prevent it by following safe sleep recommendations, while they may have a higher degree of self-efficacy regarding their ability to prevent accidental suffocation [5, 59]. In one study, mothers who reported that the sleep positioning of their infant was not up to them were more likely to intend to place their infants in the prone position [17].

Several studies have illustrated that despite parents *intending* or planning to adhere to safe sleep recommendations, their behaviors may not be consistent with that intention [15–18]. For example, one study found that fewer than half of mothers (43.7%) reported that they intended to and then actually placed their infants exclusively supine to sleep [17]. While parents may intend to practice a recommended behavior, their behavior is also influenced by additional factors, described below:

Knowledge and skills to perform the behavior

Knowledge includes basic knowledge of the safe sleep recommendations, which has been the crux of many interventions aimed at increasing adherence to recommendations [13, 39]. Knowledge also refers to an understanding of what the recommendations mean. For example, one qualitative study found that many parents did not understand that a "firm" surface meant a surface that was hard and unyielding to pressure [1]. Parents who believe that "firm" means that the sheet is tightly fit to the surface may place a pillow on top of the mattress and cover it tightly with a sheet, believing that a surface can be firm and soft at the same time [1].

Other studies have found additional misunderstandings of the safe sleep recommendations, for example, limited understanding of infant physiology, the risks of bed-sharing, and that towels and blankets placed under the infant are soft items and, thus, not recommended [45]. Thus, when providers discuss safe sleep recommendations with families, it can be helpful to begin with asking, "What do you know about safe sleep?" to help identify potential misconceptions or misunderstanding about the recommendations.

One must also have the *skills* to carry out the recommended behaviors. For example, parents may find that infants easily fall asleep in their arms, but when they try to transfer the infant to a crib, the infant wakes and cries. In this case, parents must master the skill of gently transferring the infant to the crib without waking her – for example, parents may use the technique of laying the baby in the crib and resting their hand on baby's stomach (so the baby continues to sense parent's presence). As the baby settles back to sleep, the parent can slowly remove their hand. A commonly cited reason for bed-sharing is to address crying, suggesting that added skills around soothing techniques may support parents' intentions to adhere to safe sleep recommendations [11].

Salience of the behavior

The behavior should be salient, or important, to the person and at the forefront of their thoughts [60]. For example, a parent who is sleep-deprived may decide to place the infant prone because, at that moment, sleep may be more at the forefront of his thought than a remote event such as SIDS or may use unsafe bedding that was a gift from a well-meaning relative who frequently visits (and can see if the gift is being used) [39]. *Cues to action* are internal or external factors that could trigger the health behavior or increase salience of the behavior [40]. Several studies have aimed to change infant sleep practices by providing cues to action, such as safe sleep messaging via text message reminders, in board books, or on sleep gowns or wearable blankets, or by providing recommended infant sleep surfaces such as portable cribs or travel bassinets [13, 18, 39, 61–65]. Such cues may help bring safe sleep recommendations to the forefront of parents' thoughts.

Environmental constraints

Environmental constraints are external circumstances that make a behavior "difficult to do" (requiring more energy), as opposed to "easy to do" (requiring less energy) [42, 66]. For example, lack of money to purchase a recommended sleep surface or housing constraints (such as overcrowding, limited space for a separate sleep surface, safety concerns in the home) make it difficult for a parent to comply with the recommendation of placing infant on a separate sleep surface [10, 11, 39, 67]. If an infant awakens frequently, the parent may perceive that she does not sleep as well on the back and placing her supine might require more energy than the parent has at that moment.

Additional examples of environmental constraints are current challenges or exhaustion. Although families can plan to reduce risk factors in the sleep environment, reacting to real-life stressors may undermine plans and intentions. For example, a parent may be responding to a current sleep challenge (such as infant illness or fussiness) [68–70]. Many parents have in retrospect stated that they did not know what to expect after the baby was born and thus had not planned for real-world situations or challenges, and it may be helpful for providers to set realistic expectations and discuss proactive strategies to deal with these situations should they arise. Ongoing conversations about how the baby is sleeping can help to elicit current issues; the provider can work with parents to find ways to address these issues while still maintaining safe sleep practices.

A very common environmental constraint for new parents is exhaustion. There is ample evidence of "accidental" or "unintended" bed-sharing, when parents accidentally fall asleep while caring for or feeding their infant at night [2, 20, 48, 71–74], or of placing infant in an unaccustomed prone position [75]. Parents will need strategies for keeping the infant safe when they are exhausted. If they suspect they may fall asleep while feeding, strategies could include feeding the baby on an adult bed instead of a sofa or armchair, removing dangerous items (such as loose bedding, pillows, etc.) prior to feeding the infant, or setting an alarm for 10–15 minutes to rouse themselves if they fall asleep [20].

Habit refers to the concept that repeatedly performing a behavior will lead to that behavior becoming a learned routine behavior that no longer requires prior intention or decision-making [65]. Placing an infant supine, if done repeatedly, will become a habit for parents and not something that the parent must think about doing. Following a bedtime routine that involves placing infant in his bassinet for nighttime sleep will become a habit for both parent and infant. However, if a parent has placed the infant prone several times without any adverse consequences, her experience may lead her to believe that she knows how to place the infant prone safely and thus continue to place the infant prone until it becomes a habit for both her and the infant.

Other factors are defined as demographic, personality, and individual difference variables that may be associated with behaviors but are hypothesized to have an indirect relationship via other theoretical constructs [40]. For example, beliefs and norms about infant sleep may differ among various cultural or ethnic groups, and thus, interventions should be tailored to address different audiences [11, 39].

Decision-Making About Infant Care Practices

Moon and colleagues' recent qualitative study helps to illustrate the process of parental decision-making regarding infant care [9] (Fig. 4.3). Parents (most often but not exclusively the mother) will "crowdsource" information. She will ask people whom she knows and trusts what they think that she should do; she will also go to the Internet to read what other people's opinions are. This information gathering will establish for this mother what the social norms are – "What is everyone else doing? What do others expect me to do? If I don't do this, will others judge me and think that I'm a bad mother?" This will also largely influence her attitudes about the behavior – "Is this a good idea?"

If all of the sources are consistent in their advice (further reinforcing that this is the norm and thus what she should be doing), then she will usually follow that advice. If there is inconsistency in the advice (e.g., her baby's doctor is telling her to place the baby on the back but her mother [who successfully raised six children] tells her that the baby will choke if he's on the back), then the mother has to weigh the risks and benefits of all of the advice that she has been given; she

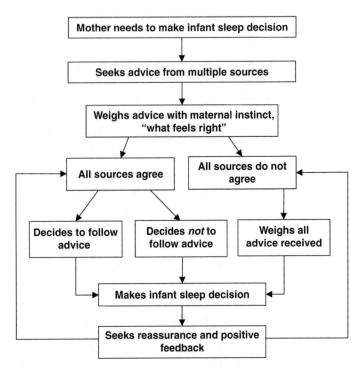

FIGURE 4.3 Path for maternal decision-making regarding infant care. (Modified from Ref. [9])

may also give more or less weight to one person's advice because of various reasons (e.g., the doctor because she is the expert on medical issues but does not know "my situation" or the grandmother because she is experienced in raising children and because she "knows my baby." She will then ultimately make a decision. When mothers describe this process, they will often refer to it as maternal instinct: "I know my baby better than anyone, and I know what is best for my baby." However, even after the mother has made a decision, she often will go back to her trusted sources for reassurance that this is really the right decision. If she gets positive feedback, she will likely continue doing what she is doing. If she gets negative feedback, she is more likely to change her behavior – often to be more consistent with what her family and friends are doing [76].

It can be difficult for mothers to make an infant care decision that is different from what others are doing. An example of this is a mother who is the first in her family to breastfeed. If she is consistently receiving negative feedback about this decision and others are trying to get her to stop breastfeeding, she may feel a great deal of pressure to give up. While she may continue to have positive attitudes about breastfeeding (e.g., it's healthier for the baby), this may not be sufficient for her to persevere in the face of constant criticism and negative feedback. Thus positive feedback is critical. If she has even one champion on her side, that can make all of the difference [77]. For some mothers, their partner is their champion that supports them and reassures them that this is the right decision. For others, it is a health-care professional or a single family member or friend who provides support.

Understanding how parents make decisions is important for health-care providers for several reasons:

- We need to realize that we are not the only sources of information for parents.
- We need to understand what others are telling parents and be able to answer the concerns (e.g., the baby will choke if she's on her back) that are often raised.
- There are multiple points in the decision-making process during which we can influence the decision-making.
- We should use social norms to help us. Remember that social norms are perceptions of reality; they may not be accurate reflections of reality. If a parent believes that "everyone places their baby on their stomach," using language indicating that this is not true may be helpful.
- We need to set realistic expectations for parents. Again, remember that social norms are perceptions; they are not reality. Parents often tell us that they had no idea that their baby was not going to sleep through the night for several months. When they are frequently asked, "Is your baby sleeping through the night yet?" they may believe that their baby is not "normal" (i.e., acting in consistency with

what the social norm is) and that they are somehow inadequate parents. Telling them in the birth hospital (or even during pregnancy) that there will be several months when the baby has to wake up every few hours to feed and that this is normal and healthy may be helpful.

- Help parents create a plan. This will increase the parents' sense of personal agency and skills:

  - What is the parents' plan for when the baby is frequently waking to feed – or is fussy – and they are exhausted? Can the parents take turns with the baby? Is there someone who can watch the baby during the day so that a parent can sleep?
  - What if the parents do not have money to buy a crib? Can we refer them to an agency that can provide a safe sleep place for the baby?
  - What does the mother need to be able to continue to breastfeed when she returns to work?

- We need to be the parents' champion to continually provide positive feedback.
- If parents feel overwhelmed by all of the "rules" that they are supposed to follow, this can decrease their sense of personal agency and their perception of their own skills to follow safe sleep guidelines. Providing small, achievable tips (e.g., try swaddling the baby to see if that will help) will be helpful.

Influencing Decision-Making

These theoretical frameworks can provide insight into how parents make decisions around infant sleep practices. To influence decision-making, providers should take a conversational approach with parents, perhaps beginning with the question, "What do you know about safe infant sleep recommendations?" followed by the question, "What questions or concerns do you have about these recommendations?" These questions can help assess what factors are most significant to the parents and can help tailor the conversation, followed by

"May I share more information about this recommendation?" which can help demonstrate respect for parents.

Even if parents do not seem to have questions, you can proactively provide guidance. For instance, if concern about choking while the baby is supine is something that you often encounter, you can address that proactively. When you do this, we would encourage you to use wording that will leverage social norms. Instead of saying, "A lot of parents worry that their baby will choke. (This implies that it is the norm to worry about.) Because you might hear this from others, I'd like to discuss this with you so that you don't worry if someone brings it up," you might say, "Most families now are placing their babies on the back. (This implies that this is the norm.) We really have not seen any problems with choking."

It is also important to provide positive feedback to parents. Remember that parents may be hearing negative feedback from others. If a parent reports that they are placing the baby on the back, give them a lot of praise and encouragement. ("I know how hard this is, and I'm so proud of you!") Several utility companies are using social norms to encourage conservation of resources and providing feedback to customers on monthly bills. The bills compare the customer's energy consumption with others in their neighborhood and provide helpful tips (e.g., "Close the curtains during summer days to decrease the need for the air conditioner" or "Do not run the water while you're brushing your teeth.") Customers whose energy consumption is higher than the norm end up decreasing their energy use. Importantly however, customers whose energy consumption is lower than the norm may increase their energy use – unless they are given positive feedback. The simple addition of a smiley face ("You used less energy this month than others in your neighborhood ☺") was enough to maintain high efficiency in those customers who were already more energy-efficient than their neighbors [78]. Thus, providing ongoing positive reinforcement to parents for their safe sleep practices is important. You may want to experiment with adding a smile sticker to the written materials that you send home with parents!

A useful resource developed by the National Center for Education in Maternal and Child Health is an online training module, *Building on Campaigns with Conversations: An individualized approach to helping families embrace safe sleep and breastfeeding* (www.ncemch.org/learning/building/), which provides information on safe sleep recommendations as well as talking points for conversations with parents. As noted, helping parents set realistic expectations for their infant's sleep and anticipate and plan for potential challenges (such as infant fussiness or illness) can help address some potential environmental constraints to adhering to safe sleep recommendations.

References

1. Ajao TI, Oden RP, Joyner BL, Moon RY. Decisions of black parents about infant bedding and sleep surfaces: a qualitative study. Pediatrics. 2011;128(3):494–502. https://doi.org/10.1542/peds.2011-0072.
2. Chu T, Hackett M, Kaur N. Exploring caregiver behavior and knowledge about unsafe sleep surfaces in infant injury death cases. Health Educ Behav. 2015;42(3):293–301. https://doi.org/10.1177/1090198114547817.
3. Gaydos LM, Blake SC, Gazmararian JA, Woodruff W, Thompson WW, Dalmida SG. Revisiting safe sleep recommendations for African-American infants: why current counseling is insufficient. Matern Child Health J. 2015;19(3):496–503. https://doi.org/10.1007/s10995-014-1530-z.
4. Herman S, Adkins M, Moon RY. Knowledge and beliefs of African-American and American Indian parents and supporters about infant safe sleep. J Community Health. 2015;40:12–9. https://doi.org/10.1007/s10900-014-9886-y.
5. Mathews A, Oden RP, Joyner BL, He J, McCarter R, Moon RY. Differences in African–American maternal self-efficacy regarding practices impacting risk for sudden infant death. J Community Health. 2016;41(2):244–9. https://doi.org/10.1007/s10900-015-0088-z.
6. Mathews A, Joyner BL, Oden RP, He J, McCarter R Jr, Moon RY. Messaging affects the behavior of African American parents

with regards to soft bedding in the infant sleep environment: a randomized controlled trial. J Pediatr. 2016;175:79–85. https://doi.org/10.1016/j.jpeds.2016.05.004.

7. Moon RY, Hauck FR. Hazardous bedding in infants' sleep environment is still common and a cause for concern. Pediatrics. 2015;135(1):178. https://doi.org/10.1542/peds.2014-3218.

8. Moon RY, Mathews A, Joyner BL, Oden RP, He J, McCarter R. Health messaging and African-American infant sleep location: a randomized controlled trial. J Community Health. 2017;42(1):1–9. https://doi.org/10.1007/s10900-016-0227-1.

9. Moon RY, Mathews A, Oden R, Carlin R. A qualitative analysis of how mothers' social networks are established and used to make infant care decisions. Clin Pediatr. 2019;58(9):985–92. https://doi.org/10.1177/0009922819845332.

10. Salm Ward TC, Doering JJ. Application of a socio-ecological model to mother-infant bedsharing. Health Educ Behav. 2014;41(6):577–89. https://doi.org/10.1177/1090198114543010.

11. Salm Ward TC. Reasons for mother-infant bedsharing: a systematic narrative synthesis of the literature and implications for future research. Matern Child Health J. 2015;19(3):675–90. https://doi.org/10.1007/s10995-014-1557-1.

12. Salm Ward TC, Ngui EM. Factors associated with bedsharing for African-American and White mothers in Wisconsin. Matern Child Health J. 2015;19(4):720–32. https://doi.org/10.1007/s10995-014-1545-5.

13. Salm Ward TC, Balfour G. Infant safe sleep interventions, 1990-2015: a review. J Community Health. 2016;41(1):180–96. https://doi.org/10.1007/s10900-015-0060-y.

14. Doering JJ, Salm Ward TC. The interface among poverty, air mattress industry trends, policy, and infant safety. Am J Public Health. 2017;107(6):945–9. https://doi.org/10.2105/AJPH.2017.303709.

15. Hooker E, Ball HL, Kelly PJ. Sleeping like a baby: attitudes and experiences of bedsharing in Northeast England. Med Anthropol. 2001;19(3):203–22. https://doi.org/10.1080/01459740.2001.9966176.

16. Hauck FR, Tanabe KO, McMurry T, Moon RY. Evaluation of bedtime basics for babies: a national crib distribution program to reduce the risk of sleep-related sudden infant deaths. J Community Health. 2015;40(3):457–63. https://doi.org/10.1007/s10900-014-9957-0.

17. Colson ER, Geller NL, Heeren T, Corwin MJ. Factors associated with choice of infant sleep position. Pediatrics. 2017;140(3):e20170596. https://doi.org/10.1542/peds.2017-0596.

18. Salm Ward TC, McClellan MM, Miller TJ, Brown S. Evaluation of a crib distribution and safe sleep educational program to reduce risk of sleep-related infant death. J Community Health. 2018;43(5):848–55. https://doi.org/10.1007/s10900-018-0493-1.

19. Ball HL, Volpe LE. Sudden infant death syndrome (SIDS) risk reduction and infant sleep location – moving the discussion forward. Soc Sci Med. 2013;79:84–91. https://doi.org/10.1016/j.socscimed.2012.03.025.

20. Doering JJ, Lim PS, Salm Ward TC, Davies WH. Prevalence of unintentional infant bedsharing. Appl Nurs Res. 2019;46:28–30. https://doi.org/10.1016/j.apnr.2019.02.003.

21. Kendall-Tackett K, Cong Z, Hale T. Factors that influence where babies sleep in the United States: the impact of feeding method, mother's race/ethnicity, partner status, employment, education, and income. Clin Lact. 2016;7(1):18–29. https://doi.org/10.1891/2158-0782.7.1.18.

22. Bronfenbrenner U. The ecology of human development. Cambridge, MA: Harvard University Press; 1979.

23. Stokols D. Establishing and maintaining healthy environments: towards a social ecology of health promotion. Am Psychol. 1992;47(1):6–22.

24. Bombard JM, Kortsmit K, Cottengim C, Johnston EO. Infant safe sleep practices in the United States. Am J Nurs. 2018;118(12):20–1. https://doi.org/10.1097/01.NAJ.0000549685.59006.ad.

25. Shapiro-Mendoza CK, Colson ER, Willinger M, Rybin DV, Camperlengo L, Corwin MJ. Trends in infant bedding use: National Infant Sleep Position Study, 1993–2010. Pediatrics. 2015;135(1):10–7. https://doi.org/10.1542/peds.2014-1793.

26. Moon RY, Carlin RF, Cornwell B, Mathews A, Oden RP, Cheng YI, et al. Implications of mothers' social networks for risky infant sleep practices. J Pediatr. 2019;212:151–8. https://doi.org/10.1016/j.jpeds.2019.05.027.

27. Rimer BK, Glanz K. Theory at a glance: a guide for health promotion practice. U.S. Department of Health and Human Services, National Cancer Institute, National Institutes of Health. NIH Publication No. 05-3896; 2005.

28. Alio AP, Richman AR, Clayton HB, Jeffers DF, Wathington DJ, Salihu HM. An ecological approach to understanding

black-white disparities in perinatal mortality. Matern Child Health J. 2010;14:557–66. https://doi.org/10.1007/s10995-009-0495-9.

29. Gamble VN. Under the shadow of Tuskegee: African Americans and health care. Am J Public Health. 1997;87(11):1773–8. https://doi.org/10.2105/ajph.87.11.1773.

30. Krieger N, Chen JT, Waterman PD, Rehkopf DH, Yin R, Coull BA. Race/ethnicity and changing US socioeconomic gradients in breast cancer incidence: California and Massachusetts, 1978–2002. Cancer Causes Control. 2006;17:217–26. https://doi.org/10.1007/s10552-005-0408-1.

31. Jones CP. Levels of racism: a theoretical framework and a gardener's tale. Am J Public Health. 2000;90(8):1212–5. https://doi.org/10.2105/ajph.90.8.1212.

32. Smedley BD, Stith AY, Nelson AR. Unequal treatment: confronting racial and ethnic disparities in health care. Institute of Medicine; 2003. https://www.nap.edu/read/10260/chapter/1#R1.

33. Acegbembo A, Tomar S, Logan H. Perceptions of racism explains the differences between blacks' and whites' level of healthcare trust. Ethn Dis. 2006;16:792–8.

34. Thomas S, Quinn S. The Tuskegee Syphilis Study, 1932–1972: implications for HIV education and AIDS risk education programs in the black community. Am J Public Health. 1991;1(11):1498–505.

35. Shavers VL, Fagan P, Jones D, Klein WMP, Boyington J, Moten C, et al. The state of research on racial/ethnic discrimination in the receipt of health care. Am J Public Health. 2012;102(5):953–66. https://doi.org/10.2105/AJPH.2012.300773.

36. Gamble VN. A legacy of distrust: African Americans and medical research. Am J Prev Med. 1993;9(Suppl 6):35–8.

37. Hwang SS, Rybin DV, Kerr SM, Heeren TC, Colson ER, Corwin MJ. Predictors of maternal trust in doctors about advice on infant care practices: the SAFE study. Acad Pediatr. 2017;17(7):762–9. https://doi.org/10.1016/j.acap.2017.03.005.

38. Hwang SS, Rybin DV, Heeren TC, Colson ER, Corwin MJ. Trust in sources of advice about infant care practices: the SAFE study. Matern Child Health J. 2016;20(9):1956–64. https://doi.org/10.1007/s10995-016-2011-3.

39. Moon RY, Hauck FR, Colson ER. Safe infant sleep interventions: what is the evidence for successful behavior change? Curr Pediatr Rev. 2016;12:67–75. https://doi.org/10.2174/1573396311166151026110148.

40. Montano DE, Kasprzyk D. Theory of reasoned action, theory of planned behavior, and the integrated behavioral model. In: Glanz K, Rimer BK, Vishwanatha KV, editors. Health behavior and health education: theory, research, and practice. 5th ed. San Francisco: Jossey-Bass; 2015. p. 95–124.

41. Fishbein M. A reasoned action approach to health promotion. Med Decis Mak. 2008;28:834–44. https://doi.org/10.1177/02729 89X08326092.

42. Fishbein M, Triandis HC, Kanfer FH, Becker M, Middlestadt SE, Eichler A. Factors influencing behavior and behavior change. In: Baum A, Revenson TA, Singer JE, editors. Handbook of health psychology. Mahwah: Lawrence Erlbaum Associates; 2001. p. 3–17.

43. Rosenstock IM. What research in motivation suggests for public health. Am J Public Health. 1960;50:295–301.

44. Hochbaum GM. Public participation in medical screening programs: a sociopsychological study. U.S. Department of Health and Human Services, United States Public Health Service. Report # 572; 1958.

45. Hirsch HM, Mullins SH, Miller BK, Aitken ME. Paternal perception of infant sleep risks and safety. Inj Epidemiol. 2018;5(Suppl 9):9. https://doi.org/10.1186/s40621-018-0140-4.

46. Roehler DR, Batra EK, Quinlan KP. Comparing the risk of sudden unexpected infant death to common causes of childhood injury death. J Pediatr. 2019;212:224–227.e5. https://doi.org/10.1016/j.jpeds.2019.05.028.

47. Fishbein M, Ajzen I. Predicting and changing behavior: the reasoned action approach. New York: Psychology Press; 2010.

48. Hauck FR, Signore C, Fein SB, Raju TN. Infant sleeping arrangements and practices during the first year of life. Pediatrics. 2008;122(2):S113. https://doi.org/10.1542/peds.2008-1315o.

49. Kendall-Tackett K, Cong Z, Hale TW. Mother-infant sleep locations and nighttime feeding behavior: U.S. data from the Survey of Mothers' Sleep and Fatigue. Clin Lact. 2010;1:27–31. https://doi.org/10.1891/215805310807011837.

50. Tomori C, Palmquist AL, Dowling S. Contested moral landscapes: negotiating breastfeeding stigma in breastmilk sharing, nighttime breastfeeding, and long-term breastfeeding in the US and the UK. Soc Sci Med. 2016;168:178–85. https://doi.org/10.1016/j.socscimed.2016.09.014.

51. Moon RY, Mathews A, Oden R, Carlin R. Mothers' perceptions of the internet and social media as sources of parenting

and health information: qualitative study. J Med Internet Res. 2019;21(7):e14289. https://doi.org/10.2196/14289.

52. Ramos KD, Youngclarke DM. Parenting advice books about child sleep: cosleeping and crying it out. Sleep. 2006;29(12):1616–23.

53. Chung M, Oden RP, Joyner BL, Sims A, Moon RY. Safe infant sleep recommendations on the internet: Let's Google it. J Pediatr. 2012;161(6):1080–4. https://doi.org/10.1016/j.jpeds.2012.06.004.

54. Sadeh A, Mindell JA, Luedtke K, Wiegand B. Sleep and sleep ecology in the first 3 years: a web-based study. J Sleep Res. 2009;18(1):60–73. https://doi.org/10.1111/j.1365-2869.2008.00699.x.

55. Galland BC, Taylor BJ, Elder DE, Herbison P. Normal sleep patterns in infants and children: a systematic review of observational studies. Sleep Med Rev. 2012;16:213–22. https://doi.org/10.1016/j.smrv.2011.06.001.

56. Hagan JF, Shaw JS, Duncan PM. Bright futures: guidelines for health supervision of infants, children, and adolescents pocket guide. 3rd ed. American Academy of Pediatrics: Elk Grove Village; 2008.

57. Bandura A. Toward a psychology of human agency. Perspect Psychol Sci. 2006;1(2):164–80.

58. Bandura A. Self-efficacy: toward a unifying theory of behavioral change. Psychol Rev. 1977;84:191–215.

59. Moon RY, Oden RP, Joyner BL, Ajao TI. Qualitative analysis of beliefs and perceptions about sudden infant death syndrome in African-American mothers: implications for safe sleep recommendations. J Pediatr. 2010;157(1):92–7. https://doi.org/10.1016/j.jpeds.2010.01.027.

60. Becker MH. The health belief model and personal health behavior. Health Educ Monogr. 1974;2:324–473.

61. Walcott RL, Salm Ward TC, Ingels JB, Llewellyn NA, Miller TJ, Corso PS. A statewide hospital-based safe infant sleep initiative: measurement of parental knowledge and behavior. J Community Health. 2018;43(3):534–42. https://doi.org/10.1007/s10900-017-0449-x.

62. Hutton J. Sleep baby safe and snug. Cincinnati: Blue Manatee Press; 2013.

63. Hutton JS, Gupta R, Gruber R, Berndsen J, DeWitt T, Ollberding NJ, et al. A randomized trial of a children's book versus brochures for safe sleep knowledge and adherence in a high-risk population. Acad Pediatr. 2017;17(8):879–86. https://doi.org/10.1016/j.acap.2017.04.018.

64. Carlin RF, Abrams A, Mathews A, Joyner BL, Oden R, McCarter R, et al. The impact of health messages on maternal decisions about infant sleep position: a randomized controlled trial. J Community Health. 2018;43(5):977–85. https://doi.org/10.1007/s10900-018-0514-0.

65. Moon RY, Hauck FR, Colson ER, Kellams AL, Geller NL, Heeren T, et al. The effect of nursing quality improvement and mobile health interventions on infant sleep practices: a randomized clinical trial. JAMA. 2017;318(4):351–9. https://doi.org/10.1001/jama.2017.8982.

66. Triandis HC. Values, attitudes, and interpersonal behavior. In: Howe HE, Page M, editors. Nebraska symposium on motivation, 1979. Lincoln: University of Nebraska Press; 1980. p. 195–259.

67. Chu T, Hackett M, Kaur N. Housing influences among sleep-related infant injury deaths in the USA. Health Promot Int. 2016;31(2):396–404. https://doi.org/10.1093/heapro/dav012.

68. Ramos KD. Intentional versus reactive co-sleeping. Sleep Res Online. 2003;5:141–7.

69. Ramos KD, Youngclarke DM, Anderson JE. Parental perceptions of sleep problems among co-sleeping and solitary sleeping children. Infant Child Dev. 2007;16(4):417–31.

70. Ramos KD. The complexity of parent-child cosleeping: researching cultural beliefs. Mothering. 2002;114:48–51.

71. Blair PS, Sidebotham P, Evason-Coombe C, Edmonds M, Heckstall-Smith EMA, Fleming P. Hazardous cosleeping environments and risk factors amenable to change: case-control study of SIDS in south west England. BMJ. 2009;339:b3666. https://doi.org/10.1136/bmj.b3666.

72. Das RR, Sankar MJ, Agarwal R, Paul VK. Is "bed sharing" beneficial and safe during infancy? A systematic review. Int J Pediatr. 2014:468538. https://doi.org/10.1155/2014/468538.

73. Lee KA, Baker FC, Newton KM, Ancoli-Israel S. The influence of reproductive status and age on women's sleep. J Women's Health. 2008;17(7):1209–14. https://doi.org/10.1089/jwh.2007.0562.

74. Smith LA, Geller NL, Kellams AL, Coslon ER, Rybin DV, Heeren T, et al. Infant sleep location and breastfeeding practices in the United States: 2011–2014. Acad Pediatr. 2016;16(6):540–9. https://doi.org/10.1016/j.acap.2016.01.021.

75. Mitchell EA, Thach BT, Thompson JMD, Williams S. Changing infants' sleep position increases risk of sudden infant death syndrome: New Zealand Cot Death Study. Arch Pediatr

Adolesc Med. 1999;153(11):1136–41. https://doi.org/10.1001/archpedi.153.11.1136.

76. Cornwell BT, Yan X, Carlin RF, Fu L, Wang J, Moon RY. Social network influences on new mothers' infant sleep adjustments. Sci Med. in press.

77. Carlin RF, Mathews A, Oden R, Moon RY. The influence of social networks and norms on breastfeeding in African American and Caucasian mothers: a qualitative study. Breastfeed Med. 2019;14(9):640–7. https://doi.org/10.1007/s10900-018-0514-0.

78. Schultz PW, Nolan JM, Cialdini RB, Goldstein NJ, Griskevicus V. The constructive, destructive, and reconstructive power of social norms. Psychol Sci. 2007;18(5):429–34. https://doi.org/10.1111/j.1467-9280.2007.01917.x.

79. Douglas R. Roehler, Erich K. Batra, Kyran P. Quinlan, (2019) Comparing the Risk of Sudden Unexpected Infant Death to Common Causes of Childhood Injury Death. The Journal of Pediatrics 212:224–227.e5.

Chapter 5
Supine (Back) Sleep Position

Bryanne N. Colvin and Eve R. Colson

Clinical Vignette

As you are rounding in the newborn nursery, you enter the postpartum room of one of your patients. The mother is present, along with the maternal grandmother. After introducing yourself, you find the infant sleeping in the bassinet on his stomach. You ask the mother, "I see your baby is sleeping on his stomach. Can you tell me about why you chose to put your baby on his stomach?"

In response, the infant's grandmother states, "I always put all my kids on their stomachs to sleep. They sleep better that way. I've done that with all my kids and they're all fine." The infant's mother then says, "I know the nurses always bring him to me on his back, but I don't really know why they do that."

Rationale: Why Supine Sleep?

Until the early 1990s, prone positioning was the most common sleep position for infants in the United States. In 1992, the American Academy of Pediatrics (AAP) released a state-

B. N. Colvin · E. R. Colson (✉)
Washington University in St. Louis School of Medicine,
St. Louis, MO, USA
e-mail: bryannecolvin@wustl.edu; eve.colson@wustl.edu

© Springer Nature Switzerland AG 2020
R. Y. Moon (ed.), *Infant Safe Sleep*,
https://doi.org/10.1007/978-3-030-47542-0_5

ment recommending supine positioning for infants as a method to prevent SIDS. This recommendation was the result of case-control studies from several countries that showed that infants placed prone were more likely to die of SIDS [1]. This led to the development of the "Back to Sleep" campaign in 1994 and an increase in supine positioning of infants in the United States. Subsequently, rates of SIDS, SUID, and overall postneonatal infant mortality decreased over the following 15 years [2, 3].

The rationale for supine positioning is supported by epidemiologic data, animal data, and human studies. Many epidemiologic studies investigating risk factors for SIDS found that both prone and side positioning increase the risk for SIDS (adjusted odds ratio (aOR) for prone 2.4–13.1, for side 2.0–3.16) [4–8], and one US study found the risk of prone (aOR 2.6, 95% CI 1.5–4.5) and side (aOR 2.0; 95% CI 1.2–3.4) to be statistically similar [6]. This is likely because infants placed on their sides can more easily roll to prone. Indeed, there may be additional risk for SIDS when infants placed on their sides are then found prone (aOR: 8.7–45.4) [4, 6]. Furthermore, infants newly placed prone after routine supine positioning are also at increased risk for SIDS (aOR 8.2–19.3) [6, 9]. Some estimate a higher population-attributable risk to side sleeping compared to prone sleeping (side 18.4%, prone 14.2%), as more infants are placed on their side to sleep [10].

The mechanism of death due to SIDS during non-supine positioning is still not fully understood. The main mechanisms that have been suggested are an increase in rebreathing expired gases, overheating, and a decrease in arousals and autonomic control. (See Chap. 2 for additional details.)

Rebreathing

The principle of "rebreathing" has long been identified as a potential mechanism for SIDS associated with prone positioning [11–13]. In this model, carbon dioxide expired from the prone infant does not freely disperse away from the infant's face and is "rebreathed" by the infant. This causes a gradual rise in the infant's carbon dioxide levels and a decrease in oxygen levels. While this does not occur in every infant placed prone, rebreathing and its effects can be significant. In one study of 56 infants, 19.6% of infants placed prone experienced desaturation events, with 25 total desaturation events documented. Three events showed desaturations to lower than 85%, and two events required interventions to terminate rebreathing [14].

While we would expect carbon dioxide to freely disperse away from an infant's face, bedding material strongly affects dispersion of gases and increases carbon dioxide accumulation around the infant, with "soft bedding" being most likely to cause accumulation [13, 15–17]. In one study from Japan, however, the authors noted that the type of bed material did not necessarily correlate with the dispersion of gases, emphasizing the importance of placing the infant supine, without any extra bedding and in a safe sleep space for every sleep [15].

The typical physiologic response to rebreathing and gradually increasing levels of carbon dioxide is a series of stereotyped behaviors. These behaviors include nuzzling into bedding, head lifts, and head repositioning. Investigations with human models have shown that nuzzling into bedding is the least effective in correcting hypoxia resulting from rebreathing, while head repositioning is the most effective. This study also demonstrated that infants unaccustomed to prone positioning displayed less effective protective behaviors than experienced infants [18]. Additional studies have shown that increasing hypercarbia generally leads to increasing states of arousal, starting with sigh breaths, then startles, then thrashing limb movements, and culminating in full arousal [19]. If the infant is unable to complete these behaviors to adjust their position away from the toxic environment, death may occur. Thus, placing infants in a supine position for sleep is the best position to ensure an effective response and prevent toxic hypercarbia and death.

Overheating

Another proposed mechanism for the harmful effects of prone positioning is the increased incidence of overheating [20–22]. The mechanism for overheating in cases of prone positioning does not appear to be related to an increase in metabolic demand, but rather a decrease in heat dissipation. This phenomenon appears to be exaggerated in low birth weight infants [23]. Additionally, overheating leads to alterations in ventilatory control, placing infants further at risk for SIDS [24, 25].

Decreased Arousal and Autonomic Control

There is extensive evidence in the literature to suggest that prone positioning decreases an infant's ability to arouse during sleep. Sleep studies of full-term infants have shown fewer spontaneous arousals during both quiet and active sleep while the infants are prone compared to when they are supine [26–29]. This phenomenon is also seen in pre-term infants and is exaggerated, even when correcting for gestational age [30–32]. Researchers conducting these studies posit that *decreased arousal may be one of the mechanisms for increased SIDS rates associated with prone positioning*. Furthermore, case-control studies of infants who underwent polysomnography and were future victims of SIDS showed decreased arousal during sleep compared to their controls [33].

Additionally, infants who are placed prone demonstrate altered autonomic function, with decreased variability in heart rate [26] as well as decreased autonomic reaction in response to head-up tilt [21, 34–36]. This change in autonomic function then leads to alterations in cerebral oxygenation during prone positioning. Investigators suggest that these changes in cerebral oxygenation may place the prone infant at increased risk for SIDS and provide an explanation for decreased arousal in these infants [35, 37, 38].

Barriers to Adherence and Strategies for Counseling Parents About Supine Sleep

Behavior theorists have found that health behaviors are driven by some predictable influences. In the theory of planned behavior, for example, Ajzen and others posit that behavior intention is strongly linked to final behavior [39], and behavior intention in turn is influenced by three main variables: attitudes, perceived social norms, and perceived control. In the case of infant sleep position, attitudes about supine sleep; perceived social norms of friends, family, and others related to supine sleep; and perceived control to make the decision, as discussed more fully below, all very much influence the choice of sleep position. Attitudes, perceived social norms, and perceived control can all present barriers to placing infants in the supine position for sleep. Many of these barriers can be effectively addressed when counseling families.

Attitudes

Researchers examining the health behaviors related to safe infant sleep have found that a number of factors strongly influence parental attitudes about supine sleeping. These attitudes often center on concerns that parents have about a given sleep position. Addressing these concerns can change attitudes which, in turn, can lead to change in behavior [40].

Both through interviews and nationally representative surveys, researchers have found that many parents do not place their infants supine to sleep because they believe infants will choke or aspirate in that position [41]. In order to address this concern, researchers using social marketing techniques and quality improvement methodologies utilized anatomic drawings to illustrate the safety of supine sleeping and explain how infants are not more likely to choke when supine (Fig. 5.1). When this issue was specifically addressed, mothers of newborns were much more likely to choose supine sleeping

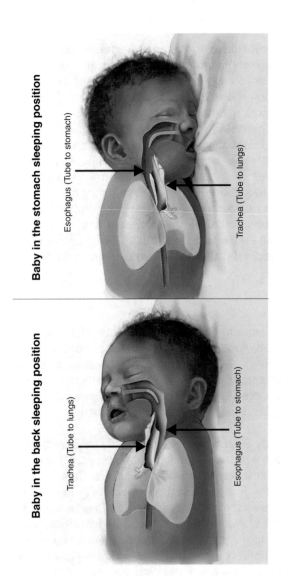

FIGURE 5.1 Infant anatomy in supine and prone position. When the infant is prone, the trachea is inferior to the esophagus. Because of gravity, regurgitated fluid will pool around the airway more readily, increasing the risk for aspiration. When the infant is supine, the trachea is superior to the esophagus. The regurgitated fluid will pool towards the esophagus, where it can be safely swallowed. (Image courtesy of the Safe to Sleep® campaign, for educational purposes only; Eunice Kennedy Shriver National Institute of Child Health and Human Development, http://www.nichd.nih.gov/sids; Safe to Sleep® is a registered trademark of the U.S. Department of Health and Human Services)

[42, 43]. (See section "Frequently Asked Questions" for specific language that can be used to explain this.)

Another common negative attitude that parents have about supine placement is the more frequent awakenings for infants in the supine position compared with prone [41]. As described above, studies have shown that this is true and, in fact, *may be protective* [26–29]. In order to address this issue, realistic expectations about normal infant sleep duration should be discussed. Parents should also be given strategies, such as use of a pacifier or swaddling, that may improve sleeping while at the same time encourage supine sleeping [44]. A pacifier can be encouraged at any time for solely formula-fed infants and, for breastfed infants, after the mother and baby are comfortable with breastfeeding, and the baby has regained birth weight and is on a positive weight gain trajectory. If swaddling is encouraged, it is critical that parents understand that the infant should always be on the back when swaddled, the hips are not so tightly swaddled as to limit movement, and they should stop swaddling their infants when the infants begin to try to roll over, which usually occurs at 2–4 months [3]. (See section "Frequently Asked Questions" for specific language that can be used to explain this.)

Parents also worry about positional plagiocephaly (asymmetry of the head shape due to sleep position) when placing their infants in the supine to sleep. This concern can be addressed by encouraging the parents to provide "tummy time" (i.e., when infants are awake and supervised while in the prone position) [3]. Such an approach will allow for development of upper body strength as well [3]. Other strategies include minimizing supine placement and maximizing upright positioning while awake and alternating the direction of the infant's body in the crib. (See section "Frequently Asked Questions" for specific language that can be used to explain this.)

Perceived Social Norms

Parents receive advice from many sources when making decisions about how to place their infants for sleep. If they are told by people whom they trust to place their infant on the stomach, they are more likely to choose that position for their baby. However, like attitudes, changing perceived social norms will, in many cases, change behavior [40].

Health-care providers are important sources of advice and can play a role in establishing perceived norms. Parents who receive advice about sleeping position from pediatricians and other health-care providers are likely to follow that advice [45]. When they do not receive any advice about sleeping position from a physician, they are less likely to place their infants supine [45]. For that reason, it is important that health-care providers tell parents to place their infants to sleep supine for every sleep.

In addition, modeling by health-care providers can have a big influence on infant sleep position. What parents see modeled in the hospital during the postpartum hospital stay or in the NICU can influence the choice they make when placing their infants to sleep at home. If a parent sees even one health-care provider placing a baby on the side or stomach, she is less likely to place her baby supine [42].

Other sources of advice include family and friends, who are quite influential with regard to choice of sleep position [45]. Mothers who are told by family or friends to place the baby on the stomach or side are more likely to do so, as they perceive that to be the prevalent ("everyone does it") and acceptable ("They will think I am a bad mother if I don't do this") behavior [46].

There are many examples of advice not consistent with recommendations found in media (such as magazines) and on the internet. One study of magazines typically read by women of childbearing age found that more than one third of pictures featured infants in the non-supine sleeping position [47]. In addition, a study of Google searches aimed at safe sleep recommendations showed as many as 10% of sites gave advice not consistent with recommendations to place infants in the supine position for sleep [48]. These sources of advice can be quite influential. In one study, compared with no advice, receiving advice from media sources to place infants supine was associated with the choice to place infants supine [45].

In addition, consistent advice is important. Those who get advice from most or all sources to place their infants in the supine position for sleep are significantly more likely to do so [45]. Therefore, it is important that health-care providers themselves advise families to place infants in the supine position for sleep and also consider other ways in which they can be change agents. Advocating for safe sleep practices in the hospital setting through quality improvement or other systematic approaches, for example, can be effective in improving consistent messaging for supine sleep [42].

Perceived Control

While attitudes and perceived norms play important roles in the decision parents make to place their infants in the supine position for sleep, ultimately they may not be able to do so if they perceive that they do not have control over the situation [39]. Lack of perceived control can occur when, for example, a family places their child in out-of-home child care. Child care providers often may place infants in the non-supine position for sleep, and approximately 20% of SIDS/SUID occur in child care settings [49–51]. Although families might express their wishes to have their infants placed in the supine position for sleep, child care providers may choose to do the opposite, depending upon their own attitudes and social norms.

Even children who receive care in their own homes by family members and other babysitters may be placed in the non-supine position for sleep. As illustrated in the case vignette, grandparents who often placed their own infants in the non-supine position may specifically want to do the same with their grandchildren [49].

Based on their home situation, parents may also perceive that they have limited choices in how to place their infants for sleep. For example, if the family situation is such that a crying infant will wake the entire family each night, a parent may choose the prone position if they believe the infant will sleep better and longer.

In summary, the supine sleep position is the safest and decreases risk of SIDS and SUID. Physiologic mechanisms that may cause increase risk in the non-supine position include rebreathing, overheating, decreased arousal, and decreased autonomic control. Despite this evidence, families do not always choose the supine position for sleep because of their attitudes; perceived social norms of friends, family, and others; as well as perceived control. Health-care providers play an important role in changing behavior by consistently modeling supine sleep practices and advising families to always place their infants on the back to sleep.

Frequently Asked Questions

What Is the Best Way to Explain the Importance of Supine Sleep to Families?

The recommendation to place infants supine to sleep changed in 1992. Researchers from countries all over the world have shown that infants are safest when placed in the supine position to sleep and are most protected from SIDS and suffocation. By placing infants in the supine position for sleep, the infants will then have clear, open air passages to their lungs. When infants are on their stomachs, they may be in a position where air cannot travel freely to their lungs. In addition, babies who sleep on their stomachs have decreased blood flow to their brain. They also sleep more deeply and so may have trouble waking up enough to get out of a situation where they don't have enough oxygen. This is why we recommend that infants be placed supine to sleep for every sleep, including naps.

Why Is Side Position Not Safe? It Seems Like a Good Compromise?

Statistically, the risk of side and prone positioning is the same. In addition, because more infants are placed on their sides compared to prone, more total infants will die of SUID when placed in this position to sleep. Side sleeping is not safe because infants can more easily roll from their sides to the prone position. That is especially unsafe because the infants are not used to sleeping in the prone position and may have trouble keeping themselves safe.

What Can I Tell Families When They Say Their Infants Will Not Sleep in the Supine Position?

Some families hear from others or may have noticed themselves that infants sleep "better" on their sides or in the prone position. It is true that many infants do sleep longer and more deeply in the prone position. However, this may be dangerous because infants may not wake up easily if they are in an unsafe situation in the prone position, such as if the infant's face is pressed against the mattress. It is important that infants wake up quickly if they are in an unsafe situation. In addition, infants should be waking frequently to feed, since their stomachs are not big enough for them to sleep more than a few hours before they need to feed again.

There are many ways for infants to sleep better in the supine position:

- Parents can consider using a white noise machine to help their babies fall asleep.
- Parents can offer a pacifier for sleep once breastfeeding has been established – i.e., the baby has regained birthweight and is continuing to gain weight. This usually happens by 2–4 weeks of age. For a solely formula-fed baby, a pacifier can be started at any time. Another advantage to this is that pacifiers have been shown to help protect infants from SIDS.
- Swaddling can help comfort infants. When swaddling infants, parents should make sure there is no loose fabric around their infants and that no fabric covers the face. They should make sure the swaddle is loose around the hips. Babies should only be on their backs when they are

swaddled. Parents should stop swaddling when their infant begins to try to roll over, which usually occurs at 2–4 months.

What Should I Tell Families When They Are Worried that Their Infant Will Choke When Sleeping in the Supine Position?

Infants choke less when they are supine than when they are prone. This is because of the way the windpipe (the trachea) and the feeding tube (the esophagus) are positioned. When infants are in the prone position, their windpipe is closer to the ground, so that when the infant spits up, gravity makes it more likely for food to enter their windpipe, causing the infant to choke. When infants are supine, their feeding tube is closer to the ground, so spit up is more likely to stay away from the windpipe, preventing the infant from choking. This is why placing infants in the supine position is safest. It is important to mention to families that they may hear the baby gagging when they spit up. This sound is due to the gag reflex, which is a sign the baby is protecting their airway, and not a sign their baby is choking. This information can be especially helpful to families when they can see an image demonstrating this point (Fig. 5.1).

What About Babies Who Have Gastroesophageal Reflux? Is It Safe for Them to Be on Their Backs?

Many infants will have reflux in the first year of life. It is important they continued to be placed flat on their back during sleep, even if they have significant reflux. Parents may express worry about their baby choking in this position, but health-care providers should reassure parents that the infant's gag reflex will protect them. Placing the baby on their stomach may even increase the risk for aspiration. Additionally, parents should be counseled against using inclined sleep surfaces, as these devices are a suffocation hazard and increase the risk of SUID. (See Chap. 10 for a more detailed discussion about gastroesophageal reflux.)

How Can I Help Families Avoid Positional Plagiocephaly in Their Infants?

Infants will spend a lot of time in the supine position in the first few months of life. There are several things families can do to help make sure their infants do not get flat or misshapen heads.

- Change the direction of the infant's body in the crib every day. For example, one day, place the infant so that her head at one end of the crib. The next day, place the infant so that her head is at the other end of the crib.
- Have "tummy time" every day. Tummy time should be when the infant is awake and supervised by an adult. Start tummy time in the first month with 1–2 minutes each time, 2–3 times per day, and as the baby gets better at it, gradually increase tummy time to 20–30 minutes each time.
- When the infant is awake, make sure that the baby is upright or in a front infant carrier, so she can have as much time out of the supine position as possible.

What Do I Tell Families When They Ask Me if the Sleep Positioner They Saw in a Store Is Safe for Their Infant?

The safest place for infants to be while they are sleeping is in the supine position. While many products claim to make unsafe sleeping positions safe for infants, these products are not necessarily tested for safety. If a product is claiming something different from what the American Academy of Pediatrics says is safe for sleep, it may not be the best and safest for the infant. (See Chaps. 8 and 9 for more information about sleep positioners and baby products.)

What Should I Tell Parents About What to Do When Their Infant Rolls Over?

Infant should be placed in the supine position for sleep until they are 1 year of age. Once infants are able to easily roll over both ways (front to back and back to front) by themselves, it is okay to leave them in that position. Families should also make sure the sleep area for infants is free of loose blankets, pillows, crib bumpers, and other toys, so that if they roll, they do not roll into something that could create a suffocation risk.

Vignette Follow-Up

While most parents will place infants on their backs to sleep, many outside factors influence and can alter this decision. When counseling parents, it is important to address the reasoning behind their decision. In this case, the family stated they put the baby on their stomach because that was what the grandmother had done in the past. Emphasizing the change in recommendations and the reasoning behind the change helps parents understand and better follow these recommendations. It is also important to address that while babies who sleep on their stomachs may sleep longer, they are at higher risk for sudden unexpected infant death, making back sleeping much safer. Offering the family tips to help their baby successfully sleep on the back, such as swaddling, pacifier use, or a white noise machine, may also help improve compliance.

Clinical Pearls

- Infants should be placed supine to sleep for every sleep.
- Frequent arousals during sleep help protect infants from SUID.

- Because of the anatomy of the esophagus and trachea, infants are less likely to aspirate while in the supine position.
- Swaddling can help infants sleep better in the supine position, but should cease when the infant begins to try to roll over, which usually occurs at 2–4 months.
- Health-care providers should discuss safe sleep with parents and other family members at every opportunity.
- Health-care providers can be change agents in their communities to spread the word that supine sleep is safest to prevent SUID deaths.

References

1. American Academy of Pediatrics AAP Task Force on infant positioning and SIDS: positioning and SIDS. Pediatrics. 1992;89(6 Pt 1):1120–6.
2. Colson ER, Rybin D, Smith LA, Colton T, Lister G, Corwin MJ. Trends and factors associated with infant sleeping position: the national infant sleep position study, 1993–2007. Arch Pediatr Adolesc Med. 2009;163(12):1122–8.
3. Moon RY, Task Force On Sudden Infant Death Syndrome. SIDS and other sleep-related infant deaths: evidence base for 2016 updated recommendations for a safe infant sleeping environment. Pediatrics. 2016;138(5):e20162940.
4. Carpenter RG, Irgens LM, Blair PS, England PD, Fleming P, Huber J, et al. Sudden unexplained infant death in 20 regions in Europe: case control study. Lancet. 2004;363(9404):185–91.
5. Hauck FR, Herman SM, Donovan M, Iyasu S, Merrick Moore C, Donoghue E, et al. Sleep environment and the risk of sudden infant death syndrome in an urban population: the Chicago Infant Mortality Study. Pediatrics. 2003;111(5 Pt 2):1207–14.
6. Li DK, Petitti DB, Willinger M, McMahon R, Odouli R, Vu H, et al. Infant sleeping position and the risk of sudden infant death syndrome in California, 1997–2000. Am J Epidemiol. 2003;157(5):446–55.
7. Pease AS, Fleming PJ, Hauck FR, Moon RY, Horne RS, L'Hoir MP, et al. Swaddling and the risk of sudden infant death syndrome: a meta-analysis. Pediatrics. 2016;137(6):e20153275.

8. Dwyer T, Ponsonby AL. Sudden infant death syndrome–insights from epidemiological research. J Epidemiol Community Health. 1992;46(2):98–102.

9. Mitchell EA, Thach BT, Thompson JM, Williams S. Changing infants' sleep position increases risk of sudden infant death syndrome. New Zealand Cot Death Study. Arch Pediatr Adolesc Med. 1999;153(11):1136–41.

10. Fleming PJ, Blair PS, Bacon C, Bensley D, Smith I, Taylor E, et al. Environment of infants during sleep and risk of the sudden infant death syndrome: results of 1993–5 case-control study for confidential inquiry into stillbirths and deaths in infancy. Confidential Enquiry into Stillbirths and Deaths Regional Coordinators and Researchers. BMJ. 1996;313(7051):191–5.

11. Bolton DP, Taylor BJ, Campbell AJ, Galland BC, Cresswell C. Rebreathing expired gases from bedding: a cause of cot death? Arch Dis Child. 1993;69(2):187–90.

12. Corbyn JA. Sudden infant death due to carbon dioxide and other pollutant accumulation at the face of a sleeping baby. Med Hypotheses. 1993;41(6):483–94.

13. Kemp JS, Thach BT. Quantifying the potential of infant bedding to limit CO_2 dispersal and factors affecting rebreathing in bedding. J Appl Physiol (1985). 1995;78(2):740–5.

14. Patel AL, Paluszynska D, Harris KA, Thach BT. Occurrence and mechanisms of sudden oxygen desaturation in infants who sleep face down. Pediatrics. 2003;111(4 Pt 1):e328–32.

15. Kanetake J, Aoki Y, Funayama M. Evaluation of rebreathing potential on bedding for infant use. Pediatr Int. 2003;45(3):284–9.

16. Kemp JS. Sudden infant death syndrome: the role of bedding revisited. J Pediatr. 1996;129(6):946–7.

17. Patel AL, Harris K, Thach BT. Inspired $CO(2)$ and $O(2)$ in sleeping infants rebreathing from bedding: relevance for sudden infant death syndrome. J Appl Physiol (1985). 2001;91(6):2537–45.

18. Paluszynska DA, Harris KA, Thach BT. Influence of sleep position experience on ability of prone-sleeping infants to escape from asphyxiating microenvironments by changing head position. Pediatrics. 2004;114(6):1634–9.

19. Lijowska AS, Reed NW, Chiodini BA, Thach BT. Sequential arousal and airway-defensive behavior of infants in asphyxial sleep environments. J Appl Physiol (1985). 1997;83(1):219–28.

20. Kleemann WJ, Schlaud M, Poets CF, Rothamel T, Troger HD. Hyperthermia in sudden infant death. Int J Legal Med. 1996;109(3):139–42.

21. Chong A, Murphy N, Matthews T. Effect of prone sleeping on circulatory control in infants. Arch Dis Child. 2000;82(3):253–6.
22. Tuffnell CS, Petersen SA, Wailoo MP. Prone sleeping infants have a reduced ability to lose heat. Early Hum Dev. 1995;43(2):109–16.
23. Ammari A, Schulze KF, Ohira-Kist K, Kashyap S, Fifer WP, Myers MM, et al. Effects of body position on thermal, cardiorespiratory and metabolic activity in low birth weight infants. Early Hum Dev. 2009;85(8):497–501.
24. Fleming PJ, Levine MR, Azaz Y, Wigfield R, Stewart AJ. Interactions between thermoregulation and the control of respiration in infants: possible relationship to sudden infant death. Acta Paediatr Suppl. 1993;82(Suppl 389):57–9.
25. Guntheroth WG, Spiers PS. Thermal stress in sudden infant death: is there an ambiguity with the rebreathing hypothesis? Pediatrics. 2001;107(4):693–8.
26. Galland BC, Reeves G, Taylor BJ, Bolton DP. Sleep position, autonomic function, and arousal. Arch Dis Child Fetal Neonatal Ed. 1998;78(3):F189–94.
27. Horne RS, Ferens D, Watts AM, Vitkovic J, Lacey B, Andrew S, et al. The prone sleeping position impairs arousability in term infants. J Pediatr. 2001;138(6):811–6.
28. Kahn A, Groswasser J, Sottiaux M, Rebuffat E, Franco P, Dramaix M. Prone or supine body position and sleep characteristics in infants. Pediatrics. 1993;91(6):1112–5.
29. Kato I, Scaillet S, Groswasser J, Montemitro E, Togari H, Lin JS, et al. Spontaneous arousability in prone and supine position in healthy infants. Sleep. 2006;29(6):785–90.
30. Ariagno RL, van Liempt S, Mirmiran M. Fewer spontaneous arousals during prone sleep in preterm infants at 1 and 3 months corrected age. J Perinatol. 2006;26(5):306–12.
31. Bhat RY, Hannam S, Pressler R, Rafferty GF, Peacock JL, Greenough A. Effect of prone and supine position on sleep, apneas, and arousal in preterm infants. Pediatrics. 2006;118(1):101–7.
32. Horne RS, Bandopadhayay P, Vitkovic J, Cranage SM, Adamson TM. Effects of age and sleeping position on arousal from sleep in preterm infants. Sleep. 2002;25(7):746–50.
33. Kato I, Franco P, Groswasser J, Scaillet S, Kelmanson I, Togari H, et al. Incomplete arousal processes in infants who were victims of sudden death. Am J Respir Crit Care Med. 2003;168(11):1298–303.

34. Tuladhar R, Harding R, Cranage SM, Adamson TM, Horne RS. Effects of sleep position, sleep state and age on heart rate responses following provoked arousal in term infants. Early Hum Dev. 2003;71(2):157–69.

35. Wong FY, Witcombe NB, Yiallourou SR, Yorkston S, Dymowski AR, Krishnan L, et al. Cerebral oxygenation is depressed during sleep in healthy term infants when they sleep prone. Pediatrics. 2011;127(3):e558–65.

36. Yiallourou SR, Walker AM, Horne RS. Prone sleeping impairs circulatory control during sleep in healthy term infants: implications for SIDS. Sleep. 2008;31(8):1139–46.

37. Fyfe KL, Yiallourou SR, Wong FY, Odoi A, Walker AM, Horne RS. Cerebral oxygenation in preterm infants. Pediatrics. 2014;134(3):435–45.

38. Wong F, Yiallourou SR, Odoi A, Browne P, Walker AM, Horne RS. Cerebrovascular control is altered in healthy term infants when they sleep prone. Sleep. 2013;36(12):1911–8.

39. Ajzen I. The theory of planned behavior. Organ Behav Hum Decis Process. 1991;50(2):179–211.

40. Moon RY, Corwin MJ, Kerr S, Heeren T, Colson E, Kellams A, et al. Mediators of improved adherence to infant safe sleep using a mobile health intervention. Pediatrics. 2019;143(5):e20182799.

41. Colson ER, Levenson S, Rybin D, Calianos C, Margolis A, Colton T, et al. Barriers to following the supine sleep recommendation among mothers at four centers for the women, infants and children program. Pediatrics. 2006;118(2):e243–50.

42. Kellams A, Parker MG, Geller NL, Moon RY, Colson ER, Drake E, et al. Todaysbaby quality improvement: safe sleep teaching and role modeling in 8 US maternity units. Pediatrics. 2017;140(5):e20171816.

43. Moon RY, Hauck FR, Colson ER, Kellams AL, Geller NL, Heeren T, et al. The effect of nursing quality improvement and mobile health interventions on infant sleep practices: a randomized clinical trial. JAMA. 2017;318(4):351–9.

44. van Sleuwen BE, Engelberts AC, Boere-Boonekamp MM, Kuis W, Schulpen TWJ, L'Hoir MP. Swaddling: a systematic review. Pediatrics. 2007;120(4):e1097–106.

45. Von Kohorn I, Corwin MJ, Rybin DV, Heeren TC, Lister G, Colson ER. Influence of prior advice and beliefs of mothers on infant sleep position. Arch Pediatr Adolesc Med. 2010;164(4):363–9.

46. Moon RY, Carlin RF, Cornwell B, Mathews A, Oden R, Cheng YI, et al. Implications of mothers' social networks for risky infant sleep practices. J Pediatr. 2019;212:151–8.
47. Joyner BL, Gill-Bailey C, Moon RY. Infant sleep environments depicted in magazines targeted to women of childbearing age. Pediatrics. 2009;124:e416.
48. Chung M, Oden RP, Joyner BL, Sims A, Moon RY. Safe infant sleep recommendations on the internet: let's Google it. J Pediatr. 2012;161:1080–4.
49. Lagon E, Moon RY, Colvin JD. Characteristics of infant deaths during sleep while under nonparental supervision. J Pediatr. 2018;197:57–62.
50. Moon RY, Biliter WM. Infant sleep position policies in licensed child care centers after back to sleep campaign. Pediatrics. 2000;106:576–80.
51. Moon RY, Weese-Mayer DE, Silvestri JM. Nighttime child care: inadequate sudden infant death syndrome risk factor knowledge, practice and policies. Pediatrics. 2003;111:795–9.

Chapter 6
Room-Sharing Without Bed-Sharing

Fern R. Hauck

Clinical Vignette

Sarah H. has an appointment for her baby, Justin, for his 2-month well-baby checkup. You ask her about how she is positioning Justin and where he sleeps at night. Sarah tells you that she places Justin on his back for every sleep. But then she sheepishly tells you that she recently started keeping Justin in bed with her and her husband as she would end up falling asleep while feeding him, even though she hadn't intended to. She is breastfeeding him and recently started back to work. She acknowledges that she knows she should not do that, but she is so exhausted and feels this is better for Justin, her husband, and her.

Background

Let's start with some definitions before we jump into this controversial topic.

- *Bed-sharing* is defined as an infant sleeping on the same surface with another person. The surface can be a bed or

F. R. Hauck (✉)
Department of Family Medicine, University of Virginia,
Charlottesville, VA, USA
e-mail: frh8e@virginia.edu

© Springer Nature Switzerland AG 2020
R. Y. Moon (ed.), *Infant Safe Sleep*,
https://doi.org/10.1007/978-3-030-47542-0_6

mattress, couch, recliner, chair, or any other surface. The person(s) sleeping with the infant is any adult or child/infant but is most often mother, father, or both parents [1].

- *Co-bedding* refers to infants, typically twins or higher-order multiples, sharing the same sleep surface.
- *Room-sharing* is defined as the infant sleeping in the parents' room but on a separate sleep surface, such as a crib or bassinet, close to the parents' bed. It is important to emphasize the protective effect of sleeping in the parents' room, not sleeping in a different room with siblings, other children, or non-parental caregivers.
- Solitary sleeping is when the infant is sleeping in a different room than the parents.

The terms *bed-sharing* and *co-sleeping* are often used interchangeably, but they do not mean the same thing. *Co-sleeping* is a practice in which infants sleep close to one or both parents, as opposed to a separate room; this close proximity, which can be on the same or different sleep surfaces, allows them to see, touch, and/or hear each other [2, 3]. Bed-sharing, therefore, is a subset of co-sleeping. The AAP recommends use of the terms bed-sharing and room-sharing, and not co-sleeping, as these are more precise terms, and their use results in less confusion [4].

As outlined in Chap. 3, the AAP 2016 Guidelines for a Safe Infant Sleeping Environment [4] state the following: *It is recommended that infants sleep in the parents' room, close to the parents' bed, but on a separate surface. The infant's crib, portable crib, play yard, or bassinet should be placed in the parents' bedroom, ideally for the first year of life, but at least for the first 6 months.* This recommendation was loosened somewhat from the previous 2011 recommendation for room-sharing, which advised to continue this practice until the infant was 1 year old, based on concerns that infants sleeping in the parents' room for that length of time could be disruptive to parental sleep.

The AAP Task Force on SIDS bases its recommendations for all the safe sleep guidelines on the published evidence; most case-control studies of SIDS risk and protective factors include infants up to 1 year of age, and therefore it is difficult to break down the recommendations to a specific age. On the other hand, 90% of SIDS deaths occur by 6 months of infant age, with the peak being 1–4 months [4]. Thus, the Task Force felt that using 6 months as the minimum age to stop room-sharing would potentially reduce the risk for the majority of infants.

The Controversy

This recommendation has been highly controversial. Breaking the controversy down, the first relates to the room-sharing part and the second to the bed-sharing part. We will start with room-sharing.

Room-Sharing Is Protective Against SIDS

The evidence from case-control studies from England, New Zealand, and Scotland supports that room-sharing reduces the risk of SIDS when compared to infants sleeping in a separate room. A study in England found that infants who slept in a separate room (e.g., solitary sleepers) compared to their parents' room had a tenfold higher risk for SIDS (adjusted odds ratio [aOR] 10.49, 95% confidence interval [CI] 4.26–25.81) [5]. The New Zealand Cot Death Study identified a 65% lower risk at last sleep for room-sharers compared with solitary sleepers (aOR 0.35, 95% CI 0.26–0.49) and a similar reduced risk for usual room-sharing [6]. A more recent New Zealand case-control study had similar findings; infants who did not room-share had an almost threefold higher risk of sudden unexpected infant death (new terminology that includes SIDS deaths) compared with room-sharers (aOR 2.77, 95% CI 1.45–5.30) [7]. A Scottish study reported a similar increased risk for sleeping in a separate room (aOR 3.26, 95% CI 1.03–10.35); this risk was found only if the parent was a smoker. However, the higher risk found in the English study was found for infants with both smoking and nonsmoking parents (P Blair, personal communication, 2016). We don't know why room-sharing is protective, but it may relate to the leading hypothesis for SIDS causation, i.e., that failure to arouse makes infants susceptible to SIDS (see Chap. 2) [8]. Room-sharing infants may have more frequent small awakenings during the night [9, 10]. Room-sharing also facilitates breastfeeding [11], which in turn confers protection against SIDS [12].

Room-Sharing May Disrupt Parents' Sleep

Concerns have been raised by parents and physicians about the recommendation to room-share. One physician noted that infants older than 6 months are more developmentally capable of vocalizing to get their parents' attention; this may lead to parental sleep deprivation and stress, especially for working mothers who have returned to work [13]. Additionally, transitioning an infant older than a year to his or her own room would be more difficult than doing it when younger than 6 months, causing greater stress to the infant. Dr. Frankel implied that the recommendation to room-share should advise this practice up to infant age of 6 months, rather than 12 months. In a commentary in the *New York Times*, Miller and Carroll wrote the following: "In our own families, when our babies were born, we both kept them in a bassinet near our beds for the first couple of months—until we couldn't take it anymore. We moved them to their own rooms because we thought it would be better for them…But we also moved them because it would be better for our own sleep" [14].

There has been some research to study the effects of room-sharing on parental and infant sleep. One study found that room-sharing mothers had more sleep disturbances than mothers who slept in a separate room [15]. They found, however, that there were no differences in sleep quality of infants room-sharing or sleeping alone.

Other studies have found that room-sharing infants have more frequent awakenings, as noted above, which may contribute to their lower risk of SIDS [9, 10]. In a longitudinal study of mother-infant pairs who had not bed-shared, at 4 months of age, infants who were early independent sleepers had longer sleep stretches (mean difference 44 minutes) and similar numbers of night awakenings [16]. At 9 months, room-sharing infants were on average sleeping 14–40 minutes less than the solitary sleepers (depending on the age of moving to their own room), and the number of night awakenings was similar. At 12 months, there were no differences in night time and daily sleep duration. These differences at earlier ages may be important to exhausted parents. However, the patterns of sleep consolidation/ longest period of sleep for the room-sharers were well within normal for infants [17], and earlier sleep consolidation may not be desirable with regard to infant arousal. Paul and colleagues found that there were differences in bedtime routines at 4 months. Bedtime routines are difficult to establish in some families and may be even more difficult in room-sharing infants. A concerning finding from this study was increased bed-sharing and exposure to soft bedding in the middle of the night for room-sharing infants.

Moon and Hauck, members of the AAP Task Force on SIDS, commented on the findings by Paul and colleagues and concluded: "We recognize that optimal parental rest is desirable…We strongly support more research, both about the physiology of infant sleep and arousal by room-sharing infants and about the consequences of room-sharing on parental and child sleep. However, the primary objective of safe sleep recommendations will always be to minimize the risk of SIDS and other sleep-related infant deaths" [18]. They further noted that other countries have similar recommendations to those of the United States; Canada, the United Kingdom, the Netherlands, and New Zealand recommend room-sharing until 6 months of age, while Australia recommends room-sharing for 6–12 months.

Guidance for Parents

Based on the evidence to date and concerns described above, here are some recommendations to help healthcare providers counsel parents about room-sharing:

- Have a discussion with parents during pregnancy, at the birth hospital stay, and at well-baby checks through at least 6 months about the recommendation to room-share (without bed-sharing). Explain in simple language that babies who room-share sleep a little less soundly and this may protect them against sleep-related infant deaths. Advise them that their own sleep may be disrupted, but reassure them that this is a short-term sacrifice.
- Try to establish bedtime routines as soon as possible, including a set bed time, feedings, etc.
- Given the higher likelihood that parents may bring the infant into bed during the night (and fall asleep) when room-sharing, parents should be advised to make sure that there are no pillows and soft bedding around the infant if they bring the infant into bed. The bed should be as "safe as possible" in advance, since most middle of the night behaviors are not planned.
- Parents can consider transitioning their infant between 6 and 12 months, especially if they are experiencing disruption of sleep that is impacting their daytime functioning.

Bed-Sharing Increases the Risk of SIDS

Bed-sharing is associated with an increased risk of SIDS. A meta-analysis of 11 studies found an almost threefold increased risk (combined OR 2.88, 95% CI 1.99–4.18) [19]. The risk was higher for smoking mothers (OR 6.27, 95% CI 3.94–9.99) and for infants <12 weeks old (OR 10.37, 95% CI 4.44–24.21). A recent New Zealand study (2012–2015) showed an even higher risk associated with bed-sharing (aOR 4.96, 95% CI 2.55–9.64) [7]. Infants exposed to both prenatal maternal smoking and bed-sharing have a markedly increased risk of sudden unexpected infant death (aOR 32.8,

95% CI 11.2–95.8) [7]. Further, bed-sharing is associated with a number of other conditions that are risk factors for SIDS, including soft bedding [20–24] and head covering [25–27]. An adult bed is not designed for infant safety and may pose additional risks for unintentional injury and death, such as asphyxia, entrapment, falls, and strangulation [28–30].

How Prevalent Is Bed-Sharing?

Bed-sharing for part or all of the infant sleep period is common. Almost half (46%) of parents of infants 8 months of age or younger participating in the National Infant Sleep Position Study (NISP) (1993–2010) reported that they shared a bed with their infant at some point in the preceding 2 weeks in the final year of the study; 13.5% reported that they usually bed-shared, compared with 6.5% reporting usual bed-sharing in 1993 [31]. A longitudinal study of infant feeding and practices found that any bed-sharing was reported by 42% of mothers at 2 weeks, 34% at 3 months, and 27% at 12 months of infant age [32]. Another study found that almost 60% of mothers of infants under 1 year of age reported bed-sharing at least once [33]. Routine bed-sharing is higher among some racial-ethnic groups including black, Hispanic, and American Indian/ Alaska Natives [34, 35]. NISP found that black mothers were over three times more likely to usually bed-share compared to white mothers. Other factors associated with higher rates of usual bed-sharing included income less than $50,000, living in the West or South (compared with the Midwest), infants younger than 16 weeks, and preterm birth. Mothers who reported that their physician advised against bed-sharing were less likely to do so (aOR 0.66, 95% CI 0.53–0.82).

Why Do Parents Bed-Share?

There are many reasons that parents bed-share, and these reasons often vary by cultural background. These include more convenience for feeding (breast or formula), to comfort a fussy or sick infant, to help the infant or mother sleep better, to promote bonding and attachment, and because it is a family tradition [32, 36]. A qualitative study of black and Hispanic mothers found that a major theme for the black participants was convenience for the purpose of being vigilant [37]. Concerns about environmental dangers, such as vermin or stray gunfire, were cited by low-income mothers as reasons to keep infants in bed with them for sleep [38].

The Controversy: Is Bed-Sharing Safe for Breastfed Infants?

Bed-sharing is associated with higher rates and prolonged duration of breastfeeding [39–41]. A longitudinal national study of infant feeding practices found that longer duration of bed-sharing was associated with a longer duration of any breastfeeding, but not exclusive breastfeeding [42]. Breastfeeding duration was longer among women who were better educated, were white, had previously breastfed, had planned to breastfeed, and had not returned to work in the first year of infant life [42]. Some experts, professional societies, and groups recommend bed-sharing to promote breastfeeding [43–48], while others do not endorse the practice because of safety concerns for the infant [8, 49, 50].

There are several circumstances that substantially increase the risk of SIDS or unintentional injury while bed-sharing: when one or both parents smoke, when the mother smoked during pregnancy, when the bed-sharer has consumed alcohol or taken medications or drugs that reduced their alertness, when bed-sharing lasts the entire night (rather than returning the infant to his/her own sleep space), and when the infant is bed-sharing with anyone who is not the infant's parent, including non-parental caregivers and other children (Table 6.1) [4, 51]. In addition, bed-sharing is particularly hazardous when it takes place on a soft surface (e.g., sofa, armchair), when there is soft bedding in the sleep space (e.g., pillows, quilts, sheepskins), and when the infant is a term normal weight infant under 4 months of age or was born preterm and/or with low birth weight (Table 6.1) [4, 51].

TABLE 6.1 Circumstances that substantially increase the risk of SIDS or unintentional injury while bed-sharing

One or both parents smoke currently
Mother smoked during pregnancy
Bed-sharer is impaired in alertness (alcohol, medications, drugs)
Bed-sharing on a soft surface (sofa, armchair)
Soft bedding in sleep environment (pillows, blankets, sheepskins)
Bed-sharing with non-parental caregivers, other children
Bed-sharing for entire night
Infant who was born preterm and/or low birth weight
Term infant under 4 months of age

The evidence, however, is somewhat conflicting regarding the risk of bed-sharing among infants under less hazardous conditions, namely, those who are breastfed and whose parents are nonsmokers and have not consumed alcohol, medications, or drugs that reduce alertness. The AAP Technical Report, which provides the evidence base for the 2016 Recommendations for a Safe Infant Sleeping Environment, describes two sets of analyses that evaluated bed-sharing under these less hazardous conditions [8]. The first was an analysis of 19 studies from 9 datasets in the United Kingdom, Europe, and Australasia to determine the risk of SIDS from bed-sharing when an infant was breastfed and the parents did not smoke and had not taken alcohol or illicit drugs. The adjusted odds ratio for breastfed bed-sharing infants without these other factors was 2.7 (95% CI 1.4–5.3) [52]. The risk was highest in the first 2 weeks of life (aOR 8.3, 95% CI 3.7–18.6) and in the first 3 months of life (aOR 5.1, 95% CI 2.3–11.4). There was inadequate power to assess the risk of SIDS for infants over 3 months of age. This study has been criticized for imputing the large amount of missing data for parental alcohol and drug use, although the methods used to impute the missing data were appropriate.

The second analysis was from two case-control studies in England (1993–1996 and 2003–2006); the adjusted OR for bed-sharing in the absence of parental alcohol or tobacco use was 1.1 (95% CI 0.6–2.9) [53]. For infants under the age of 98 days, the OR was 1.6 (95% CI 0.96–2.7). These results were independent of feeding method. The methods have been criticized for the choice of controls, which may have biased the results towards the null [8].

Both studies are limited by small sample size for the no-other-risk factors group. The AAP concluded, with the consultation of an independent statistician, that both studies have strengths and weaknesses and should be interpreted with caution. While they appear to contradict each other, their data do not support definitive differences and do not support a definitive conclusion that bed-sharing in the youngest age group is safe, even under less hazardous circumstances [8].

Guidance for Parents

Based on the evidence to date and concerns and controversies described above, here are some recommendations to help healthcare providers counsel parents about bed-sharing (note, a separate chapter is devoted to breastfeeding and bed-sharing and is not discussed here; see Chap. 7):

- Have a discussion with parents during pregnancy, at the birth hospital stay, and at well-baby checks through 12 months about the recommendation to avoid bed-sharing. All medical personnel should provide a consistent message to avoid parental confusion.
- This subject, perhaps being the most sensitive and controversial of the safe sleep recommendations, requires sensitivity on the part of the practitioner and an approach that is a dialogue rather than telling the parents what they should and should not do.

    - Since this approach may take longer than the time available for patient anticipatory guidance, providers may want to take a team approach, by training other office staff, such as nurses, to discuss bed-sharing with parents.

- Use open-ended questions and anticipate that parents may be considering bed-sharing or may have bed-shared with their other children. Ask specifically about their plans or thoughts about bed-sharing and prior experiences (either personally or among their family and friends) to establish what is culturally or socially considered the norm for them. If they say they plan to bed-share, without judgment or bias (providers may have bias for or against bed-sharing, often based on their own experience), ask them to explain more about that to better understand their reasons as well as any anticipated barriers they may have to room-sharing without bed-sharing, such as lack of access to a crib.
- If they lack access to a crib, refer them to a local agency that can provide a crib. Most communities have crib donation programs to provide cribs at no cost to eligible parents.
- Reflect on their reasons for anticipating or currently bed-sharing and address these issues. Explain the evidence for the recommendation not to bed-share in language appropriate to the level of education of the parents. Offer alternative measures, such as swaddling (if age appropriate), for an infant who has trouble settling for sleep on a separate surface.
- Advise parents that infants brought into bed for feeding or comforting should be returned to their own crib or bassinet. It is less hazardous to feed the baby in bed than on a couch or armchair should the parent fall asleep. Anticipate that falling asleep is common, so when the baby is brought into bed, all soft bedding materials should be removed from around the baby.
- If parents are adamant about bed-sharing, be sure to remind them that there are certain conditions that are very hazardous (see Table 6.2) and strongly discourage them from bed-sharing if any apply to them [8].

TABLE 6.2 High-risk bed-sharing situations

The sleep surface is soft or has a risk of entrapment, such as a waterbed, old mattress, couch, or armchair

The bed-sharer is a current smoker or if the mother smoked during pregnancy

The bed-sharer is impaired in his or her alertness or ability to arouse because of fatigue or sedating medications or substances

Infants under 4 months of age

Infants who were preterm or low birth weight

The bed-sharer is not the infant's parent. This includes the infant's siblings and other relatives

- Have materials available in your office/clinic about the safe to sleep guidelines and websites that parents can access directly for information. The Resources section at the end of this book provides a listing of some helpful websites.

Vignette Follow-Up

This is something you hear pretty often, and it is challenging to convince tired mothers, especially those who are breast-feeding, to avoid bed-sharing for the night. Start out by sympathizing and telling her that this is a challenging situation and you are there to help offer some support and guidance. Ask Sarah what she knows about the risks of bed-sharing. Then ask what she sees as the benefits. If her risks list is fairly short, you can provide a little more "data" and point out that Justin is in the peak age range for SIDS and that we want to lower the risk of SIDS as much as possible. Some ways other moms have dealt with this include using a play yard, bassinet, or bedside co-sleeper which, when placed next to Sarah's bed, makes it easier for her to move Justin into her bed to nurse him without even getting out of bed. She could ask her husband to help, by putting Justin back in his sleep space after feedings if Sarah falls asleep. They can take turns setting their phone alarms in case they fall asleep. Suggest that she talk to family or friends who breastfed without bed-sharing, to see how they did it. Being intentional about limiting hazards in her bed is also important: keep Justin away from pillows and blankets while nursing, so if Sarah does unintentionally fall asleep, Justin's sleep space is clear of potentially asphyxiating hazards. Check back with Sarah to see what she thinks about these suggestions and let her know that you and your office staff are available to support her.

Clinical Pearls

- The safest place for a baby to sleep is in a crib, bassinet, or play yard in the parents' room, close to the parents' bed. This allows for easy access to the infant for feeding and monitoring.
- Increased arousals during the night may be why room-sharing is protective.
- Behaviors in the middle of the night are often unplanned. Therefore, if there is a chance that the parent may fall asleep while feeding the baby, the adult bed should be proactively prepared to be as safe as possible: firm (hard) mattress with no pillows or blankets.
- High-risk bed-sharing situations (Table 6.2) should be avoided.

References

1. Hauck FR, Herman SM, Donovan M, Iyasu S, Merrick MC, Donoghue E, et al. Sleep environment and the risk of sudden infant death syndrome in an urban population: the Chicago Infant Mortality Study. Pediatrics. 2003;111(5):1207–14.
2. McKenna JJ, Thoman EB, Anders TF, Sadeh A, Schechtman VL, Glotzbach SF. Infant-parent co-sleeping in an evolution-ary perspective: implications for understanding infant sleep

development and the sudden infant death syndrome. Sleep. 1993;16(3):263–82.

3. McKenna JJ, Ball HL, Gettler LT. Mother-infant cosleeping, breastfeeding and sudden infant death syndrome: what biological anthropology has discovered about normal infant sleep and pediatric sleep medicine. Am J Physical Anthropol. 2007;Suppl 45:133–61. https://doi.org/10.1002/ajpa.20736.

4. Task Force on Sudden Infant Death Syndrome. SIDS and other sleep-related infant deaths: updated 2016 recommendations for a safe infant sleeping environment. Pediatrics. 2016;138(5):e20162938. https://doi.org/10.1542/peds.2016-2938.

5. Blair PS, Fleming PJ, Smith IJ, Platt MW, Young J, Nadin P, et al. Babies sleeping with parents; case-control study of factors influencing the risk of the sudden infant death syndrome. BMJ: Br Med J. 1999;319:1457–62.

6. Mitchell EA. Smoking: the next major and modifiable risk factor. In: Rognum TO, editor. Sudden infant death syndrome. New trends in the nineties. Oslo: Scandinavian University Press; 1995. p. 114–8.

7. Mitchell EA, Thompson JM, Zuccollo J, MacFarlane M, Taylor B, Elder D, et al. The combination of bed sharing and maternal smoking leads to a greatly increased risk of sudden unexpected death in infancy: the New Zealand SUDI Nationwide Case Control Study. N Z Med J. 2017;130(1456):52–64.

8. Moon RY. SIDS and other sleep-related infant deaths: evidence base for 2016 updated recommendations for a safe infant sleeping environment. Pediatrics. 2016;138(5):e20162940. https://doi.org/10.1542/peds.2016-2940.

9. Mao A, Burnham MM, Goodlin-Jones BL, Gaylor EE, Anders TF. A comparison of the sleep-wake patterns of cosleeping and solitary-sleeping infants. Child Psychiatry Hum Dev. 2004;35(2):95–105. https://doi.org/10.1007/s10578-004-1879-0.

10. Mindell JA, Sadeh A, Kohyama J, How TH. Parental behaviors and sleep outcomes in infants and toddlers: a cross-cultural comparison. Sleep Med. 2010;11(4):393–9. https://doi.org/10.1016/j.sleep.2009.11.011.

11. Smith LA, Geller NL, Kellams AL, Colson ER, Rybin DV, Heeren T, et al. Infant sleep location and breastfeeding practices in the United States, 2011–2014. Acad Pediatr. 2016;16(6):540–9. https://doi.org/10.1016/j.acap.2016.01.021.

12. Hauck FR, Thompson JM, Tanabe KO, Moon RY, Vennemann MM. Breastfeeding and reduced risk of sudden infant death syn-

drome: a meta-analysis. Pediatrics. 2011;128(1):103–10. https://doi.org/10.1542/peds.2010-3000.

13. Frankel LA. RE: room-sharing until 12 months. Pediatrics. 2017;139(3):e20164132B. e20164132B [pii].

14. Miller CC, Carroll AE. Should your baby really sleep in the same room as you? New York Times. 2016 November 4. p. 2.

15. Volkovich E, Ben-Zion H, Karny D, Meiri G, Tikotzky L. Sleep patterns of co-sleeping and solitary sleeping infants and mothers: a longitudinal study. Sleep Med. 2015;16(11):1305–12. https://doi.org/10.1016/j.sleep.2015.08.016.

16. Paul IM, Hohman EE, Loken E, Savage JS, Anzman-Frasca S, Carper P, et al. Mother-infant room-sharing and sleep outcomes in the INSIGHT study. Pediatrics. 2017;140(1):e20170122. https://doi.org/10.1542/peds.2017-0122.

17. Galland BC, Taylor BJ, Elder DE, Herbison P. Normal sleep patterns in infants and children: a systematic review of observational studies. Sleep Med Rev. 2012;16(3):213–22. https://doi.org/10.1016/j.smrv.2011.06.001.

18. Moon RY, Hauck FR. Are there long-term consequences of room-sharing during infancy? Pediatrics. 2017;140(1):e20171323. https://doi.org/10.1542/peds.2017-1323.

19. Vennemann MM, Hense HW, Bajanowski T, Blair PS, Complojer C, Moon RY, et al. Bed sharing and the risk of sudden infant death syndrome: can we resolve the debate? J Pediatr. 2012;160(1):44–8.e2. https://doi.org/10.1016/j.jpeds.2011.06.052.

20. Scheers NJ, Dayton M, Kemp JS. Sudden infant death with external airways covered. Arch Pediatr Adolesc Med. 1998;152: 540–7.

21. Unger B, Kemp JS, Wilkins D, Psara R, Ledbetter T, Graham M, et al. Racial disparity and modifiable risk factors among infants dying suddenly and unexpectedly. Pediatrics. 2003;111(2):E127–E31.

22. Kemp JS, Unger B, Wilkins D, Psara RM, Ledbetter TL, Graham MA, et al. Unsafe sleep practices and an analysis of bedsharing among infants dying suddenly and unexpectedly: results of a four-year, populationbased, death-scene investigation study of sudden infant death syndrome and related deaths. Pediatrics. 2000;106(3):e41.

23. Drago DA, Dannenberg AL. Infant mechanical suffocation deaths in the United States, 1980–1997. Pediatrics. 1999;103(5):e59–66.

24. Fu LY, Moon RY, Hauck FR. Bed sharing among black infants and sudden infant death syndrome: interactions with other

known risk factors. Acad Pediatr. 2010;10(6):376–82. https://doi.org/10.1016/j.acap.2010.09.001.

25. Blair PS, Mitchell EA, Heckstall-Smith EM, Fleming PJ. Head covering – a major modifiable risk factor for sudden infant death syndrome: a systematic review. Arch Dis Child. 2008;93(9):778–83. https://doi.org/10.1136/adc.2007.136366.

26. Baddock SA, Galland BC, Bolton DPG, Williams SM, Taylor BJ. Differences in infant and parent behaviors during routine bed sharing compared with cot sleeping in the home setting. Pediatrics. 2006;117(5):1599–607.

27. Ball H. Airway covering during bed-sharing. Child Care Health Dev. 2009;35(5):728–37. https://doi.org/10.1111/j.1365-2214.2009.00979.x.

28. Ostfeld BM, Perl H, Esposito L, Hempstead K, Hinnen R, Sandler A, et al. Sleep environment, positional, lifestyle, and demographic characteristics associated with bed sharing in sudden infant death syndrome cases: a population-based study. Pediatrics. 2006;118(5):2051–9. 118/5/2051 [pii]. https://doi.org/10.1542/peds.2006-0176.

29. Scheers NJ, Rutherford GW, Kemp JS. Where should infants sleep? A comparison of risk for suffocation of infants sleeping in cribs, adult beds, and other sleeping locations. Pediatrics. 2003;112(4):883–9.

30. Erck Lambert AB, Parks SE, Cottengim C, Faulkner M, Hauck FR, Shapiro-Mendoza CK. Sleep-related infant suffocation deaths attributable to soft bedding, overlay, and wedging. Pediatrics. 2019;143(5):e20183408. https://doi.org/10.1542/peds.2018-3408.

31. Colson ER, Willinger M, Rybin D, Heeren T, Smith LA, Lister G, et al. Trends and factors associated with infant bed sharing, 1993–2010: the National Infant Sleep Position Study. JAMA Pediatr. 2013;167(11):1032–7. https://doi.org/10.1001/jamapediatrics.2013.2560.

32. Hauck FR, Signore C, Fein SB, Raju TN. Infant sleeping arrangements and practices during the first year of life. Pediatrics. 2008;122(Suppl 2):S113–20. https://doi.org/10.1542/peds.2008-1315o.

33. Kendall-Tackett K, Cong Z, Hale TW. Mother-infant sleep locations and nighttime feeding behavior: U.S. data from the Survey of Mothers' Sleep and Fatigue. Clin Lact. 2010;1(1):27–31.

34. Lahr MB, Rosenberg KD, Lapidus JA. Maternal-infant bedsharing: risk factors for bedsharing in a population-based survey

of new mothers and implications for SIDS risk reduction. Matern Child Health J. 2007;11:277–86. https://doi.org/10.1007/s10995-006-0166-z.

35. Fu LY, Colson ER, Corwin MJ, Moon RY. Infant sleep location: associated maternal and infant characteristics with sudden infant death syndrome prevention recommendations. J Pediatr. 2008;153(4):503–8. https://doi.org/10.1016/j.jpeds.2008.05.004.

36. Salm Ward TC, Balfour GM. infant safe sleep interventions, 1990–2015: a review. J Community Health. 2016;41(1):180–96. https://doi.org/10.1007/s10900-015-0060-y.

37. Mathews AA, Joyner BL, Oden RP, Alamo I, Moon RY. Comparison of infant sleep practices in African-American and US Hispanic families: implications for sleep-related infant death. J Immigr Minor Health. 2015;17(3):834–42. https://doi.org/10.1007/s10903-014-0016-9.

38. Joyner BL, Oden R, Ajao TI, Moon R. Where should my baby sleep? A qualitative study of African-American infant sleep location decisions. J Natl Med Assoc. 2010;102:881–9.

39. Horsley T, Clifford T, Barrowman N, Bennett S, Yazdi F, Sampson M, et al. Benefits and harms associated with the practice of bed sharing: a systematic review. Arch Pediatr Adolesc Med. 2007;161:237–45.

40. Blair PS, Heron J, Fleming PJ. Relationship between bed sharing and breastfeeding: longitudinal, population-based analysis. Pediatrics. 2010;126(5):e1119–26. https://doi.org/10.1542/peds.2010-1277.

41. McKenna JJ, Mosko SS, Richard CA. Bedsharing promotes breastfeeding. Pediatrics. 1997;100(2):214–9.

42. Huang Y, Hauck FR, Signore C, Yu A, Raju TNK, Huang TT-K, et al. Influence of bedsharing activity on breastfeeding duration among US mothers. JAMA Pediatr. 2013;167(11):1038–44. https://doi.org/10.1001/jamapediatrics.2013.2632.

43. Ball HL. Breastfeeding, bed-sharing, and infant sleep. Birth. 2003;30(3):181–8.

44. McKenna JJ, McDade T. Why babies should never sleep alone: a review of the co-sleeping controversy in relation to SIDS, bedsharing and breast feeding. Paediatr Respir Rev. 2005;6(2):134–52.

45. Bartick M, Smith LJ. Speaking out on safe sleep: evidence-based infant sleep recommendations. Breastfeed Med. 2014. https://doi.org/10.1089/bfm.2014.0113.

46. Should I sleep with my baby? La Leche League, International. https://www.llli.org/breastfeeding-info/sleep-bedshare/. Accessed 15 Oct 2019.

47. Academy of Breastfeeding Medicine Protocol Committee. ABM clinical protocol #6: guideline on co-sleeping and breastfeeding. Revision, March 2008. Breastfeed Med. 2008;3(1):38–43. https://doi.org/10.1089/bfm.2007.9979.

48. Co-Sleeping and SIDS: a guide for health professionals. UNICEF. 2019. https://www.unicef.org.uk/babyfriendly/wp-content/uploads/sites/2/2016/07/Co-sleeping-and-SIDS-A-Guide-for-Health-Professionals.pdf. Accessed 29 Oct 2019.

49. Ways to reduce the risk of SIDS and other sleep-related causes of infant death. National Institute of Child Health and Human Development. https://safetosleep.nichd.nih.gov/safesleepbasics/risk/reduce. Accessed 15 Oct 2019.

50. Parents and caregivers: learn what parents and caregivers can do to help babies sleep safely. Centers for Disease Control and Prevention. https://www.cdc.gov/sids/Parents-Caregivers.htm. Accessed 15 Oct 2019.

51. Moon RY, Hauck FR. Risk factors and theories. In: Duncan JR, Byard RW, editors. SIDS sudden infant and early childhood death: the past, the present and the future. Adelaide: University of Adelaide Press; 2018.

52. Carpenter R, McGarvey C, Mitchell EA, Tappin DM, Vennemann MM, Smuk M, et al. Bed sharing when parents do not smoke: is there a risk of SIDS? An individual level analysis of five major case-control studies. BMJ Open. 2013;3(5):e002299. https://doi.org/10.1136/bmjopen-2012-002299.

53. Blair PS, Sidebotham P, Pease A, Fleming PJ. Bed-sharing in the absence of hazardous circumstances: is there a risk of sudden infant death syndrome? An analysis from two case-control studies conducted in the UK. PloS One. 2014;9(9):e107799. https://doi.org/10.1371/journal.pone.0107799.

Chapter 7
Breastfeeding Without Bed-Sharing

Ann Kellams

Clinical Vignettes

Scenario 1

Carolyn is a 31-year-old accountant and non-smoker with an 8-week-old son, Ryan, who was born at 39 weeks' gestation. She has been back at work for 2 weeks. Ryan is still waking up multiple times at night and sometimes has a difficult time settling down after a feeding. Carolyn is exhausted. She has fallen asleep while feeding and holding him in the padded chair in their room, often startling awake and fearing she might drop him. She is drowsy and not herself at work. Her friend suggested that she bring Ryan into her bed so he can feed whenever he wants and she can get some rest.

Scenario 2

Deanna is 28 years old, and Jackie is her third child who was born 3 weeks ago at 36 weeks' gestation. She has a 4- and a 2-year-old son as well. She is essentially a single mom as her husband is deployed with the military. She smokes ½ pack of cigarettes per day and cannot imagine stopping smoking, especially at such a stressful time. Jackie's pediatrician has never inquired about her sleep location but has advised

A. Kellams (✉)
University of Virginia, Department of Pediatrics,
Charlottesville, VA, USA
e-mail: ALK9C@hscmail.mcc.virginia.edu

© Springer Nature Switzerland AG 2020
R. Y. Moon (ed.), *Infant Safe Sleep*,
https://doi.org/10.1007/978-3-030-47542-0_7

against bed-sharing, and Deanna has nodded and said "okay" and has not mentioned that she sometimes shares a bed with Jackie as a "survival strategy."

The Importance of Breastfeeding

Breastmilk is the ideal source of nutrition and protection for infants. It changes with every stage of development and contains antibodies and infection-fighting substances that are specific to the environment that the mother and baby share. It promotes gut maturity and the development of a healthy microbiome and contains anti-inflammatory substances that help build tolerance rather than sensitivity to common allergens. Infants who breastfeed have significantly lower risk of diarrheal and lower respiratory infections, SIDS, childhood asthma and obesity, and the development of diabetes [1]. In addition, mothers who breastfeed their infants have lower rates of breast cancer and ovarian cancer, type II diabetes, and heart disease [2, 3]. For these and many other health benefits, the AAP as well as the Centers for Disease Control and Prevention and other health and scientific organizations recommend 6 months of exclusive breastfeeding for all infants for whom there is not a contraindication, followed by breastfeeding and complementary foods until the infant is at least 1 year of age [4, 5]. It is estimated that, if 90% of infants in the USA were exclusively breastfed for 6 months, three billion dollars in healthcare costs (79% maternal) would be saved and there would be >2500 fewer maternal and >700 fewer infant deaths per year [2].

Rates of Breastfeeding in the USA

In the 1970s and 1980s, breastfeeding initiation rates in the USA were as low as ~25%. Since the early 1990s, given the growing emphasis on the importance of breastfeeding, rates have been steadily rising, with most recent data showing that

83.2% of US mothers are initiating breastfeeding [6]. Despite these relatively high initiation rates, however, there is a steep drop-off, with more than 2/3 of mothers not achieving their personal breastfeeding goals [7], only 25% making it to 6 months of exclusive breastfeeding and only 35% still breastfeeding at 1 year of age [6]. Huge disparities exist, with non-Hispanic black women breastfeeding at much lower rates than non-Hispanic white women and women of lower education and socioeconomic status breastfeeding less than those of higher education and incomes [8].

Rates of Bed-Sharing in the USA

Despite the AAP recommendation for all infants to room-share but not bed-share [9], a substantial portion of mothers in the USA reports bed-sharing at least some of the time [10–12]. A study using telephone surveys examined national trends in bed-sharing between 1993 and 2010 and showed an increase in bed-sharing, particularly for African American and Hispanic women. In that study, 40% of non-Hispanic black women reported that they usually shared a bed with their infant [11]. Smith and colleagues found that 21% of a nationally representative sample reported bed-sharing for all or part of the night [12]. While Back-to-Sleep campaigns have clearly changed infant sleep position practices, the message to room-share without bed-sharing has not been as successful, perhaps indicating a need to nuance or somehow change the message [13].

Breastfeeding Is Protective against SIDS

Recent meta-analyses have demonstrated that breastfeeding has a protective effect against SIDS. In a multivariate meta-analysis of 18 studies, the adjusted odds ratio (aOR) for any breastfeeding vs. no breastfeeding was 0.55 [95% CI 0.44–0.69] [14]. Another more recent analysis of individual-level data from eight case-control studies showed that any breast-feeding for at least 2 months duration was protective and that the effect was stronger with increasing duration (aOR 2–4 months: 0.60 [95% CI 0.44, 0.82]; 4–6 months aOR 0.40 [95% CI 0.26, 0.63]; and > 6 months aOR 0.36 [95% CI 0.22, 0.61]). Breastfeeding did not have to be exclusive to confer this protective effect. Essentially, any breastfeeding duration of at least 2 months halved the rate of SIDS [15].

Additionally, there are data to suggest that breastfeeding mothers and babies who share a bed sleep differently and breastfeed more frequently than mothers and babies who sleep in close proximity but not on the same surface. More frequent feeds contribute to maintenance of a full milk supply by providing more frequent signaling to the mother's body. Bed-sharing infants arouse more frequently, which may offer some protection against SUID, with less time in stage 3 and 4 deep sleep. Mothers who bed-share show increased maternal touching and looking at their infant; they also have faster and more frequent maternal responses [16].

Bed-Sharing Promotes Breastfeeding

Recent longitudinal data has shown that bed-sharing promotes breastfeeding [10], and data from the USA and across the globe show a dose-dependent relationship, in that women who report more bed-sharing breastfeed for longer durations. This holds true for both any and exclusive breastfeeding. It is not known whether this is cause and effect, but the association is strong across multiple studies [17, 18].

How to Talk About this with Families

Advice from doctors about both breastfeeding and bed-sharing is important. Smith and colleagues showed that mothers who received advice to breastfeed and to room-share without bed-sharing were more likely to do both [12].

However, 20% of new mothers in that survey reported that they did not receive any advice from physicians about safe sleep or breastfeeding, indicating that we have a long way to go to support these mothers. Further complicating things is the seemingly conflicting advice that families often receive from both breastfeeding and safe sleep advocates. Helping families navigate the varying recommendations and come up with a plan that is right for them to achieve both goals of successful breastfeeding and safe sleep is a priority. It turns out that the recommendations from some of the major breast-feeding and bed-sharing advocates have more in common with the AAP safe sleep recommendations than not. In particular, there is agreement that breastfeeding is recommended to help lower the risk of SUID and that bed-sharing should be avoided in particularly hazardous situations, including soft mattresses or the presence of soft bedding, in the presence of cigarette smoke exposure, when a parent is under the influence of a sedating medication or substance, and when the infant is sick or premature (see Table 7.1). In addition, there is no doubt that sharing a couch or a sofa as a sleep surface poses a huge risk. In other words, for feedings when the parent is exhausted, it is better that they occur on a firm, flat adult mattress that is free of soft bedding instead of a couch, sofa, or armchair. Below is a framework for having these conversations with families in a way that helps them have all of the current information and feel empowered to

TABLE 7.1 AAP: circumstances that substantially increase the risk of SUID while bed-sharing

Infant younger than 4 months
With a current smoker or maternal smoking during pregnancy
With someone impaired by sedating medications or substances
With anyone who is not the infant's parent
On a soft surface such as a waterbed, old mattress, sofa, couch, or armchair
With soft bedding such as pillows or blankets

make informed decisions that are right for them. Having these conversations can help the family plan for safe sleeping and feeding spaces in case they fall asleep with the infant.

Guidance for Parents

1. *Rather than starting with what they "should" or "shouldn't" do, begin the conversation by asking parents about their plans for feeding the baby and where the baby will sleep.* Inquire about the reasoning behind those decisions and what they think the barriers might be for them to room-share without bed-sharing. Listen with a nonjudgmental stance, using an attitude of inquiry and curiosity, so that they will feel comfortable sharing. Use open-ended questions.

   Examples:

   "What are your plans for where your baby will sleep?"
       "Tell me a little bit about how the night times are going?"
       "Where/how do you start out the night? And where/how do you end up?"
       "What do you do when you are exhausted and at risk of falling asleep and baby needs to be fed?"
       "Are you familiar with the recommendation to room-share but not bed-share?"

2. *Do a risk assessment for SIDS/SUID for that particular baby*

   (See Table 7.1)
       Is the infant younger than 4 months of age?
       Is there a current smoker in the household, or was the baby exposed to maternal smoking during pregnancy?
       Is the parent taking or using any medications or substances that could affect arousability?
       Is the infant sleeping with anyone other than a parent?

What is the sleep surface like? Is it an adult bed? A water-bed? A couch or armchair, etc.? What items are present in the sleep surface, i.e., comforters, pillows, stuffed animals, etc.?

3. *Tailor education and family-centered plans to the particular situation and risk assessment and teach SIDS/SUID risk reduction strategies*

   Use nuanced conversation strategies such as motivational interviewing techniques that have been proven to help with other behavioral/lifestyle changes.

   Examples:

   "You mentioned that she sleeps with you on the couch because she 'likes to be held.' Have you tried any other strategies for helping her sleep? We worry most about couches or sofas."

   "Do you have a sense of why we recommend that baby has their own separate sleep surface?"

   "Have you thought about trying to soothe or feed her in your bed, with the crib or bassinet close by so you can put her back in her own space? That would probably be safer than falling asleep with her on a couch or sofa due to the risk of suffocation" [13, 19, 20].

   "One thing we worry about with babies exposed to cigarette smoke is that they may not have the same ability to handle lower oxygen levels. I wonder if, for her, it might be especially important to figure out a way for her to sleep near you but not in the bed with you?"

   "What do you think are some things that would help you be successful in the middle of the night when she is feeding frequently?"

4. *Empower families and encourage self-efficacy, given all of the information and their current situation, to choose the practices and plans that will work best for them.*

   Example:

   "I want to make sure you have all of the information about what the recommendations are and why so you can make the best choices for you and your baby/family."

5. *Discuss strategies for keeping the baby safe when frequent feedings are required and the parent is exhausted.*

Example:

Think of the letter "F" for "falling asleep while feeding" when thinking about safety for feeding when you are at risk of falling asleep (Table 7.2).

See Fig. 7.1.

6. *Spend the most time counseling those families whose infants are at the highest risk.*
7. *Review strategies to maximize parental rest and encourage parental self-care:*

   (a) Discuss the mindset of a 24-hour sleep schedule and the importance of napping/resting during the day whenever possible and self-care for the parents and especially the mother.
   (b) Line up family and friend support and/or home nursing or postpartum doula services to help with other infant caring tasks and household duties.

TABLE 7.2 Suggestions for a planned feeding space when the parent is at risk of falling asleep [21]

Face up

Flat, firm bed/mattress (NOT a couch, sofa, or armchair)

Free of objects and soft bedding

Feeding only breastmilk

Free of anyone other than a parent

"Fashioned" infant sleep space nearby for after feeding (i.e., crib or bassinet right next to your bed)

"Fully aware" parent who is non-drowsy and not under the influence of sedating medications or substances

Fully vaccinated

Fresh air—Avoid overheating and no one that smokes in the bed or environment

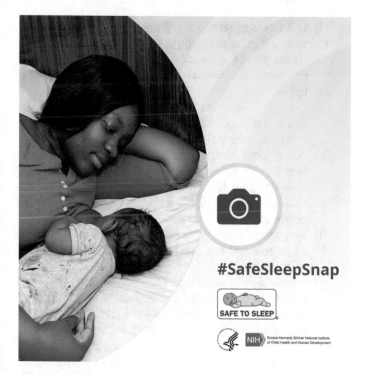

FIGURE 7.1 Breastfeeding in an adult bed from the NICHD #SafeSleepSnap campaign. (Available for free download at: https://www.flickr.com/photos/nichd/48918388683/in/album-72157654071312421/)

(c) Allow baby to feed "on cue" or "cluster feed" (i.e., responsive feeding), as this frequent feeding will often be followed by a longer sleep period.

(d) With each feeding, suggest burping baby or changing the diaper or doing some infant massage techniques, as needed to help rouse the baby to keep feeding so that at least one breast is fully drained.

(e) Recommend gentle breast compression during feedings to stimulate milk letdown and increased infant suckling and hand expression after feedings to maximize signal to the breasts and intake of infant.

(f) Recommend setting up "feeding stations" for mother with water, snacks, diaper changing materials, burp cloths, etc., so infant care can be bundled and mother can take advantage of times when baby is not feeding to rest.

(g) Line up adults, care partners, etc. to snuggle, hold, and watch baby after breastfeeding so mother can perform self-care and rest.

(h) Normalize feelings of difficulty, exhaustion, and worry that this phase will never end and a sense of feeling overwhelmed. Help mothers to have realistic expectations of what it is like to be postpartum and care for a newborn.

(i) Emphasize that the mother has also been "born" into a new role and that it is normal to go through a period of adjustment.

(j) Screen for Perinatal Mood and Anxiety Disorders (PMADs) using a validated tool such as the Edinburgh Postpartum Depression Scale at each scheduled clinical encounter in the first year after birth.

Available at: https://www.aap.org/en-us/advocacy-and-policy/aap-health-initiatives/practicing-safety/Documents/Postnatal%20Depression%20Scale.pdf

(k) When the mother is awake and not breastfeeding, suggest prioritizing activities or tasks that make her "feel good" and help her feel like herself—e.g., talking with family or friends, resting even if not sleeping, going outside, and taking an uninterrupted shower.

(l) Point mother to evidence-based resources and websites for information about parenting, breastfeeding, and safe sleep such as the CDC.gov or HealthyChildren.org or the Academy of Breastfeeding Medicine at bfmed.org (see Resources section at end of book for additional resources).

(m) Consider an online or virtual support group, or once the mother feels up to leaving the house, look into local mother's groups or breastfeeding groups or support groups.

8. *Become skilled in assessment of effectiveness and adequacy of breastfeeding and perform this assessment at every encounter with the infant or dyad:*

   (a) Baby wakes easily and often to feed and then is settled for a time after feedings.
   (b) Baby is feeding at least eight to ten times in 24 hours (on the baby's schedule, not by the clock).
   (c) Mother is offering the breast with every feeding cue — turning head, opening mouth, sucking fingers, rooting, stirring, and not waiting for crying which is a late sign of hunger.
   (d) Mother is not having nipple compression or soreness during or in between feedings (indicating a problem with positioning which can limit the amount of signaling and milk transfer).
   (e) Swallows are audible: for infants in the first 2–3 days, swallows at least every four to five suckles; for older infants, periods during the feeding of swallowing with almost every suckle.
   (f) Infant is having at least one bowel movement per day for the first 5 days and at least one wet diaper for every day of age, with six to eight wet diapers/day by age 5 days.
   (g) Stools have changed over to yellow/green, seedy stools by day 5.
   (h) Mother is producing ounces of milk by day 4–5.
   (i) After the nadir of weight at day 3–4, infant is gaining at least 15–30 grams/day on average.
   (j) On physical exam, infant is active, mucous membranes are moist, and skin turgor is normal.

9. *Discuss ways to help calm/soothe infant at times when infant is not feeding.*

   (a) Swaddling for infants less than 2 months of age with a thin cotton blanket, with no material above the shoulder line and completely tucked around infant.
   (b) Rhythmic swaying or gentle bouncing or patting.

TABLE 7.3 Components of safe positioning for the newborn while skin-to-skin [22]

1.	Infant's face can be seen.
2.	Infant's head is in "sniffing" position.
3.	Infant's nose and mouth are not covered.
4.	Infant's head is turned to one side.
5.	Infant's neck is straight, not bent.
6.	Infant's shoulders and chest face mother.
7.	Infant's legs are flexed.
8.	Infant's back is covered with blankets.
9.	Mother-infant dyad is monitored continuously by staff in the delivery environment and regularly on the postpartum unit.
10.	When mother wants to sleep, infant is placed in bassinet or with another support person who is awake and alert.

(c) Changing positions—example infant facing out or in arms on his or her side or walking outside or into a different room.

(d) Soothing talking, singing, music, or "shushing."

(e) Placing baby skin-to-skin with an awake and alert parent or caregiver following the AAP components for safe skin-to-skin care (Table 7.3).

(f) Offering an upside-down pinkie finger or a pacifier (for infants for whom breastfeeding is well-established) for suckling. Breastfeeding is considered well-established when the infant is above birthweight, mother has a full milk supply, and infant cues to feed and latches effectively and comfortably each feeding. This usually occurs by 2 to 4 weeks of age.

Frequently Asked Questions

What do I do if I discover a mother is bed-sharing?

As in the scenarios above, first of all, it is important to inquire about infant care practices in a nonjudgmental way so that families feel comfortable being honest. Acknowledge that having a newborn is hard and that there are multiple competing priorities including breastfeeding, safe sleep, and the need for parental rest. Discuss the particular risk factors that the baby has and ideas for how the family could reduce the risk of SUID. For example, instead of feeding in a chair or sofa, discuss what a safer, planned feeding space might look like with a firm adult mattress, no thick/fluffy pillows or blankets, and a bassinette or crib right next to the bed for the baby to sleep in between feedings.

Is bed-sharing always unsafe?

The absolute safest place for a baby to sleep is in their own sleep space in close proximity to the mother as, even in a planned nighttime feeding space, there is still a potential risk of overlying. The studies looking at bed-sharing for low-risk mothers are not definitive, with one showing no significant increased risk in the absence of hazardous bed-sharing risk factors and another showing an increased risk in those infants with no other risk factors who were less than 4 months of age [23, 24]. In the AAP Evidence Base for 2016 Updated Recommendations for a Safe Infant Sleeping Environment [25], with the assistance of an independent biostatistician, they concluded: "There is some evidence of an increased risk in the no-other-risk-factor setting, in particular in the youngest age groups." The bottom line is that bed-sharing, even in the absence of other hazardous risk factors, may pose some risk even for infants with no other risk factors, particularly for infants less than 4 months of age.

How do I advise a mother who reports she is falling asleep while feeding her baby?

First of all, you can acknowledge that parenting a young infant is exhausting and let her know that you understand how this can happen. Talk with her about a planned feeding space that is on a flat, firm adult mattress without soft bedding and with a crib or bassinet nearby to place the baby in when the parent is ready to go back to sleep. (See Table 7.2.)

Is it possible to breastfeed successfully without bed-sharing?

Yes! Many women room-share without bed-sharing and successfully breastfeed. It takes a commitment, planning, and perseverance, just like any other important lifestyle and behavioral goal. The strategies outlined above will likely help, as will receiving advice from physicians to strive for both, and planning nighttime sleep and feeding spaces to minimize disruption of sleep will help ease the burden of frequent night feedings and maximize safety.

What do safe sleep and breastfeeding recommendations have in common?

Breastfeeding is protective against SIDS and provides optimal nutrition, protection, and health benefits for mothers and babies. For breastfeeding and for safe sleep, it is important that the mother and infant are in close proximity to allow for frequent feedings and maximize the mother's ability to respond to her infant. Both recommendations strive to keep babies safe and help them thrive. All of the recommendations agree that there are particularly hazardous circumstances for which bed-sharing would not be recommended (see Table 7.1).

Vignette Follow-Up

Scenario 1

First, assess how effectively Ryan is feeding—Is his growth appropriate? Is Carolyn having any breast soreness? Does at least the first breast feel "emptied" after he feeds? You could perhaps empathize with her about how hard it is to be a new parent, return to work, care for a young infant, etc. It might be effective to highlight the shared goal of her wanting to sleep and also breastfeed and keep her baby safe. You could ask her if she has ever tried breastfeeding side-lying and discuss with her the recommendation to room-share but not bed-share and the "why" behind it—concern for accidental suffocation/strangulation. Then, consider talking about what a safe feeding space might look like and review the "F"s of feeding, for example, in her bed with the baby's bassinet just beside her so she can put him back in his own sleep space when they're done with feeding and removing fluffy, soft pillows and blankets, etc. (see Table 7.2).

Scenario 2

First, your practice could include inquiring at each well check about how the night times are going for Jackie and Deanna and express empathy with being a tired new parent. A good lead-in question might be to ask "Where does Jackie usually start off the night, and where does she end up?" so you can identify if she bed-shares. You could also ask about where and how she usually accomplishes feedings when she is exhausted. If you find out she is bed-sharing and/or falling asleep while feeding Jackie, you could talk about what a safe feeding space might look like and review the "F"s of feeding, e.g., in her bed with baby's bassinette just beside so she can put him back in his own sleep space and removing fluffy, soft pillows and blankets, etc. (see Table 7.1). You could then also strategize with her about what things might help her take care of herself during this stressful time.

Clinical Pearls

1. Breastfeeding and room-sharing without bed-sharing are not mutually exclusive.
2. Use nonjudgmental language and open-ended questions when talking with families about bed-sharing and breastfeeding.
3. Identify families for whom bed-sharing may be particularly dangerous, e.g., prematurity, couch/sofa, etc.

Brainstorm with the family about the best feeding plan for when they are at risk of falling asleep (see Table 7.2).
4. Become skilled at assessing breastfeeding and help families ensure that baby is effectively feeding each time to help lessen the burden of frequent night feedings/wakenings.s.
5. Encourage parental self-care and review strategies to help families navigate the early days of caring for a newborn.

Bibliography

1. Chowdhury R, Sinha B, Sankar MJ, Taneja S, Bhandari N, Rollins N, et al. Breastfeeding and maternal health outcomes: a systematic review and meta-analysis. Acta Paediatr. 2015;104(467):96–113.
2. Bartick MC, Schwarz EB, Green BD, Jegier BJ, Reinhold AG, Colaizy TT, et al. Suboptimal breastfeeding in the United States: Maternal and pediatric health outcomes and costs. Matern Child Nutr. 2017;13(1):1–13. https://onlinelibrary.wiley.com/doi/epdf/10.1111/mcn.12366.
3. Stuebe A. Associations among lactation, maternal carbohydrate metabolism, and cardiovascular health. Clin Obstet Gynecol. 2015;58(4):827–39.
4. Breastfeeding and the use of human milk. Pediatrics. 2012;129(3):e827–41.
5. Recommendations and Benefits | Nutrition | CDC [Internet]. [cited 2019 Oct 31]. Available from: https://www.cdc.gov/nutrition/infantandtoddlernutrition/breastfeeding/recommendations-benefits.html.
6. Breastfeeding Report Cards | Breastfeeding | CDC [Internet]. [cited 2017 Nov 1]. Available from: https://www.cdc.gov/breastfeeding/data/reportcard.htm.
7. Perrine CG, Scanlon KS, Li R, Odom E, Grummer-Strawn LM. Baby-friendly hospital practices and meeting exclusive breastfeeding intention. Pediatrics. 2012;130(1):54–60.
8. Beauregard JL, Hamner HC, Chen J, Avila-Rodriguez W, Elam-Evans LD, Perrine CG. Racial disparities in breastfeeding initiation and duration among U.S. infants born in 2015. MMWR Morb Mortal Wkly Rep. 2019;68(34):745–8.
9. Task Force on Sudden Infant Death Syndrome. SIDS and Other Sleep-Related Infant Deaths: Updated 2016

Recommendations for a Safe Infant Sleeping Environment. Pediatrics. 2016;138(5). https://pediatrics.aappublications.org/task_force_on_sudden_infant_death_syndrome.

10. Huang Y, Hauck FR, Signore C, Yu A, Raju TNK, Huang TT-K, et al. Influence of bedsharing activity on breastfeeding duration among US mothers. JAMA Pediatr. 2013;167(11):1038–44.

11. Colson ER, Willinger M, Rybin D, Heeren T, Smith LA, Lister G, et al. Trends and factors associated with infant bed sharing, 1993-2010: the National Infant Sleep Position Study. JAMA Pediatr. 2013;167(11):1032–7.

12. Smith LA, Geller NL, Kellams AL, Colson ER, Rybin DV, Heeren T, et al. Infant sleep location and breastfeeding practices in the United States, 2011–2014. Acad Pediatr. 2016;16(6):540–9.

13. Altfeld S, Peacock N, Rowe HL, Massino J, Garland C, Smith S, et al. Moving beyond "abstinence-only" messaging to reduce sleep-related infant deaths. J Pediatr. 2017;189:207–12.

14. Hauck FR, Thompson JMD, Tanabe KO, Moon RY, Vennemann MM. Breastfeeding and reduced risk of sudden infant death syndrome: a meta-analysis. Pediatrics. 2011;128(1):103–10.

15. Thompson JMD, Tanabe K, Moon RY, Mitchell EA, McGarvey C, Tappin D, et al. Duration of breastfeeding and risk of SIDS: an individual participant data meta-analysis. Pediatrics. 2017; 140(5). https://pubmed.ncbi.nlm.nih.gov/29084835/.

16. Baddock SA, Purnell MT, Blair PS, Pease AS, Elder DE, Galland BC. The influence of bed-sharing on infant physiology, breastfeeding and behaviour: a systematic review. Sleep Med Rev. 2019;43:106–17.

17. Ball HL, Howel D, Bryant A, Best E, Russell C, Ward-Platt M. Bed-sharing by breastfeeding mothers: who bed-shares and what is the relationship with breastfeeding duration? Acta Paediatr. 2016;105(6):628–34.

18. Blair PS, Heron J, Fleming PJ. Relationship between bed sharing and breastfeeding: longitudinal, population-based analysis. Pediatrics. 2010;126(5):e1119–26.

19. Resnicow K, McMaster F. Motivational interviewing: moving from why to how with autonomy support. Int J Behav Nutr Phys Act. 2012;9:19.

20. Rubak S, Sandbaek A, Lauritzen T, Christensen B. Motivational interviewing: a systematic review and meta-analysis. Br J Gen Pract. 2005;55(513):305–12.

21. Kellams A. Balancing safe sleep and other recommendations for newborns. Neonatology for primary care, 2nd ed. Textbook. 2020. p. 285–99.
22. Feldman-Winter L, Goldsmith JP, Committee on Fetus and Newborn, Task Force on Sudden Infant Death Syndrome. Safe sleep and skin-to-skin care in the neonatal period for healthy term newborns. Pediatrics. 2016;138(3). https://pubmed.ncbi.nlm.nih.gov/27550975/.
23. Blair PS, Sidebotham P, Pease A, Fleming PJ. Bed-sharing in the absence of hazardous circumstances: is there a risk of sudden infant death syndrome? An analysis from two case-control studies conducted in the UK. PLoS One. 2014;9(9):e107799.
24. Carpenter R, McGarvey C, Mitchell EA, Tappin DM, Vennemann MM, Smuk M, et al. Bed sharing when parents do not smoke: is there a risk of SIDS? An individual level analysis of five major case-control studies. BMJ Open. 2013;3(5). https://bmjopen.bmj.com/content/3/5/e002299.citation-tools.
25. Moon RY, Task Force on Sudden Infant Death Syndrome. SIDS and Other Sleep-Related Infant Deaths: Evidence Base for 2016 Updated recommendations for a safe infant sleeping environment. Pediatrics 2016;138(5):e20162940.

Chapter 8
Use of Soft Bedding and Other Soft Surfaces

Rebecca Carlin

Clinical Vignette

You are seeing Avery for her 2-week weight check. She was born full term after an uncomplicated pregnancy and has overall been doing well since coming home from the well-baby nursery. She is exclusively breastfed and surpassed her birth weight at today's visit. She lives at home with her mother, father, and dog. No one in the home smokes tobacco. You ask her parents where and how she is sleeping and they tell you she has a bassinet in their room and she is being placed on her back. Her parents' only concern at today's visit is that she is a noisy breather when she sleeps. They ask to show you a video so you can hear it. On the video, the baby sounds slightly congested and does not appear to be struggling; however, when you look at the screen, you note that she is placed in the bassinet on a U-shaped pillow and she has loose muslin blanket over her. How do you counsel Avery's parents?

R. Carlin (✉)
Columbia University, New York, NY, USA
e-mail: rfc2101@cumc.columbia.edu

© Springer Nature Switzerland AG 2020
R. Y. Moon (ed.), *Infant Safe Sleep*,
https://doi.org/10.1007/978-3-030-47542-0_8

Introduction

The use of soft or loose bedding has long been known to significantly increase the risk of SIDS. The Chicago Infant Mortality Study found that regardless of sleep position, infants placed to sleep on a soft surface had five times the risk of SIDS, while those using pillows or found to have their face or head covered by soft bedding had almost three times the risk of SIDS [1]. Additionally, the combination of soft bedding and prone position increased the risk of SIDS by 21-fold [1]. While loose bedding and soft sleep surfaces may play a role in any sudden and unexpected infant death, their role is even more prominent in cases coded as accidental suffocation or strangulation in bed (ASSB). A recent analysis of the population-based sudden unexpected infant death case registry from 2011 to 2014 found that 69% of deaths classified as ASSB were attributable to soft bedding [2].

The AAP safe sleep recommendations include A-level recommendations to use a firm sleep surface for infant sleep and to eliminate loose bedding soft objects from the infant's sleep area, as these can increase the risk of SIDS, suffocation, entrapment, and strangulation [3]. However, while the rates of reported non-supine sleeping have fallen in recent decades, soft bedding usage remains prevalent, with one survey finding that 1/3 of mothers report infants have soft bedding in their sleep environment [4]. In order to appropriately counsel families and help them adhere with these recommendations, it is important for healthcare providers to understand the soft bedding and unsafe sleep environments most commonly used and the barriers to adherence with the recommendations.

To simplify this recommendation, "soft or loose bedding" should be defined as anything in the infant's sleep environment other than a tight fitted sheet and what the infant is wearing (i.e., clothing, wearable blankets, swaddle sacks). Common examples of soft or loose bedding are listed in Table 8.1. Certain potential sleep surfaces also carry inherent risks for suffocation, often because a non-breathable surface (e.g., cushioned chair or soft mattress) can conform to the

TABLE 8.1 Specific common soft bedding items to avoid	
	Loose blankets or sheets
	Stuffed animals
	Crib bumpers
	Wedges and positioning devices, including U-shaped pillows
	Pillows
	Soft mattress pads

TABLE 8.2 Specific common sleep surfaces to avoid

Couch or sofa
Cushioned chair
Soft mattress (including memory foam, air mattresses, and waterbeds)
Any inclined (more than 10 degrees from horizontal) sleep surface
Car seat
Swing
Crib, bassinet, or play yard with an ill-fitting mattress

infant's face, or because the infant is positioned (e.g., on an inclined sleep surface or in a car seat) in such a way that allows the airway to be otherwise compromised. The most common of these surfaces are listed in Table 8.2.

When discussing safe sleep with new parents, it is helpful to consider how they generally understand SIDS and pertinent risk factors, particularly soft or loose bedding. Although parents whose infants are at high risk for sleep-related deaths often feel they have no control over whether SIDS happens or not (and thus see no point in following safe sleep guidelines), qualitative data indicate that they believe that suffocation can be avoided [5]. One study found a significant decrease in the proportion of African-American women who used soft bedding when standard safe sleep educational materials replaced the word "SIDS" with "SIDS and suffocation." [6] *Therefore, providers discussing safe sleep with parents may find it beneficial to include accidental suffocation and strangulation as reasons to follow safe sleep guidelines.*

Importance of a Firm Sleep Surface

The AAP recommends all infants sleep on a firm, flat surface. While parents often assume their child will be most comfortable sleeping on a soft, plush surface similar to many adult beds, such a surface is both unnecessary for infant sleep and poses potential hazards to infants. Indeed, two surveys of ASSB deaths found that the mattress was the obstructing object in approximately 20% of sleep-related suffocations [2, 7]. As the AAP recommendations detail, the danger in soft surfaces, including memory foam, lies in the fact that it can create a pocket or indentation that can increase the risk of rebreathing and suffocation should an infant be placed or roll into the prone position. Even without a clear indentation, infants are likely to struggle for leverage on a softer surface. Should an infant be placed or roll into the prone position, it will be more difficult for her to push up on her arms to either lift her head or roll onto her back on a soft surface than a firm one, due to the give of the mattress; this increases the risk for rebreathing or suffocation. For this same reason, the AAP warns against placing any soft bedding under a sleeping infant, even if the soft materials are covered by a sheet [3]. Such materials mimic the danger of a soft mattress as is illustrated in Fig. 8.1.

To standardize the safety of mattresses, the Consumer Product Safety Commission (CPSC) specifies that full-size crib mattresses be ≤ 6 inches in thickness [8]. Mattresses should feel firm, such that when pressure is applied to both the center and perimeter, there should be quick recoil and no mark left at the pressure point. Although there is a standard size for full-size mattresses, the same does not apply for non-full-size mattresses (e.g., for bassinets, larger- or smaller-sized

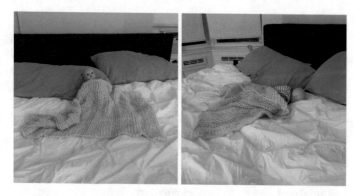

Figure 8.1 Hypothetical infant death scene based on actual death scene investigative photos. The left frame shows the infant was placed to sleep against a pillow, covered in blankets on an adult bed. The right frame shows the infant rolled supine with his face down in the pillow. (Permission Rebecca Carlin)

cribs, play yards, and other soft-sided sleepers). Thus, parents should be counseled to only use a mattress that tightly fits the crib, bassinet, or play yard [3].

Although some mattresses and sleep devices advertise that they are composed of materials that can lead to a decreased risk of rebreathing, this has never been scientifically proven. Thus, they should be considered unsafe if they do not meet CPSC specifications for thickness and firmness. The AAP notes that there is no disadvantage to these products if they meet these safety specifications.

Common Barriers to Adherence

Over 50% of ASSBs occurs on a shared sleep surface [2]. Given that adult mattresses rarely meet crib standards for firmness, the desire to bed-share is a common barrier to adherence. (For more information on this topic, please see Chap. 6.) Parents may also place infants on a soft surface within their own crib, bassinet, play yard, or similar surface, because they perceive the crib to be uncomfortable for the infant in the absence of these soft items [9]. Unless this perception is altered, it can be difficult to convince families to change this behavior. In some cases, alternative sleep locations, such as couches, mattresses on the floor, or other soft surfaces, are chosen due to space constraints and limited resources for an appropriate sleep surface.

Counseling Parents on a Firm Sleep Surface

The average age for ASSB is 3.76 months [7], making counseling about sleep surface particularly important beginning from the early newborn period. As with all counseling, when talking to parents about the importance of a firm sleep surface, it is important to identify their specific barriers to adherence so they may be appropriately addressed. When parents are utilizing a soft, shared sleep surface because of a desire to bed-share, counseling techniques outlined in Chap. 6 should be the first line. In the case of parents whose primary reason for choosing a soft sleep surface is infant comfort, parents should be advised that evidence shows infants are more secure and safe on a firm surface. In order to help parents understand the risk inherent in placing infants on such surfaces, it can be helpful to demonstrate with the infant how he lifts his head and why that would be more difficult on a soft surface than a firm one.

It is also important to clarify the parents' understanding of a "firm" surface. A qualitative study found that many parents did not understand that a firm surface was to be hard or unyielding. The most common understanding was that a firm surface was one over which the sheet was wrapped tightly; thus, parents believed that a surface could be both firm and soft if the parent placed a pillow on top of the mattress and then wrapped it tightly with a sheet [9].

Parents should be counseled on the CPSC safety standards for firm sleep surfaces described above. Additionally, the AAP recommends finding a mattress designed for the specific product in use in order to prevent wedging that can occur with ill-fitting mattresses and discussed further below.

Local organizations can often provide free or low-cost safe sleep surfaces for infants whose families have limited financial resources (see Resources at end of the book).

Sofas and Cushioned Chairs

When perusing baby pictures, one can often find adorable photos of infants sleeping on a parent on the couch. Unfortunately though, as picturesque as this may appear, it is an extremely dangerous sleep environment (see Chap. 1). Studies have shown a 49–67-fold increased risk of sleep-related deaths on a sofa/couch, compared to other sleep surfaces such as a crib. US surveillance data between 2004 and 2012 revealed that almost 13% of sleep-related infant deaths occurred on a sofa [10]. Sofas, couches, and cushioned chairs are inherently risky sleep surfaces, as they are typically soft, curved surfaces; infants are easily lodged between the cushions, and it is difficult, particularly for young infants, to extract themselves prior to suffocation (Fig. 8.2). The risk on sofas in particular is increased further by the fact that they are a frequent site for an adult and infant to fall asleep together; the infant slips off the adult (often a parent's)'s chest and is wedged between cushions. Infants who die on sofas are more likely to be found in a different position and on a different surface than they were initially [10]. These factors indicate that the behavior was likely not planned.

Common Barriers to Adherence

Most parents who fall asleep on the sofa with their infant often do not intend to do so. It is likely that the parent was feeding, burping, trying to soothe, or just snuggling and then fell asleep. As discussed in Chaps. 6 and 7, caring for an infant is exhausting, and thus it is not unusual for caregivers to accidentally fall asleep holding their infant, particularly when breastfeeding.

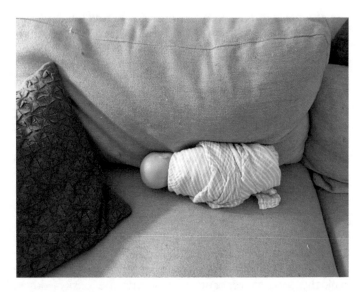

FIGURE 8.2 Hypothetical death scene based on death scene investigation in which an infant was placed swaddled on a couch to sleep. The infant became wedged between the pillow and the back of the couch. (Permission Rebecca Carlin)

Parents in small apartments and resource-limited settings may also report there is no other place for them to sit or sleep other than the sofa or a cushioned chair.

Counseling Families About Sofas and Cushioned Chairs

It is important that families understand the potential hazard of sofas and cushioned chairs for sleep and that they be counseled to plan appropriately when sitting down on one with their infant. Parents should be discouraged from feeding or holding infants on such surfaces, particularly for nighttime feedings, when they themselves are so tired that they may fall asleep. It is much safer to feed the infant on the parents' bed than on a sofa or cushioned chair. Thus, parents should be encouraged to create a feeding plan that does not include sofas or cushioned chairs when they are tired and that specifically identifies a safe surface (e.g., a play yard) nearby in which to place the infant if the parent becomes sleepy, as it is easier to enact a behavior that has already been thought through. Parents should also be encouraged to talk to other household members about the danger of infants sleeping on sofas or chairs so that they too can move the infant if they see a caregiver asleep with her.

In cases where resources and space are limited, it is critical to know the resources available in your community for portable safe sleep surfaces that can be used in small spaces and then folded up when the infant is awake.

Inclined Sleepers and Positioners

Gastroesophageal reflux (GER) affects 50% of infants under 3 months [11]. Standard reflux precautions often include holding infants upright for 30 minutes after feeding. Historically, providers have recommended placing infants on an incline to sleep for a similar gravitational benefit to prevent further spit up. There are both products, including car seats, bouncers, swings, and inclined sleepers, that can place the infants directly into an inclined position, and positioners, such as wedges and U-shaped pillows on which one can place an infant to create the incline. However, studies looking at placing children supine on an incline to decrease GER have in fact demonstrated increased rather than decreased GER symptoms [12]. The North American Society for Pediatric Gastroenterology, Hepatology, and Nutrition (NASPGHAN) and the European Society for Pediatric Gastroenterology, Hepatology, and Nutrition (ESPGHAN) concur with the AAPs advice that even infants with gastroesophageal reflux should sleep supine on a flat surface. (For more details about safe sleep for infants with GER, please see Chap. 10.)

After a series of reported deaths in inclined sleepers, the CPSC commissioned a supplemental report on inclined sleepers and recalled several models in 2019 and 2020. As part of the report, CPSC hired a mechanical engineer to look at the safety of inclined sleepers. The Mannen report had several key findings, including that more muscle strength is required for infants to remain on an incline, and thus, if infants roll to prone, they may be too fatigued to lift their head or roll back [13]. Additionally, because muscle synergies are different in the inclined position, it may be easier to roll from supine to prone on an incline, and if an infant rolls to the prone position on an incline, she is likely unaccustomed to the prone position. Prone lying in an inclined sleeper also results in lower oxygen saturation and thus is higher risk. Similar to other studies [14, 15], Mannen found that, even when the infant is properly strapped to the surface, the incline places the infant in a position where her head may fall forward and increase her risk of apnea and SIDS. The report concluded that it was unsafe for infants to sleep on any surface with an incline greater than 10 degrees from the horizontal [13].

Positioners are pillows, foam, or other materials that are placed directly under or next to an infant in order to keep the infant in a designated position. These are particularly dangerous, as infants can slide or roll off of them, resulting in entrapment between the positioner and either the mattress or a wall or suffocation against the positioner [2, 7]. V-shaped adult pillows have been implicated as a particularly high-risk object in the past [16], and newer U-shaped pillows, designed for assistance with breastfeeding and tummy time, seem to pose a similar hazard [17]. As is shown in Fig. 8.3, infants can easily slide off such objects and flip to the unaccustomed prone position. The risk of entrapment or wedging increases if the positioner is on a soft surface, making it harder for the infant to reposition if he slides or rolls off the device.

Barriers to Adherence

Avoidance of inclined sleepers and positioners can be a particularly difficult recommendation for parents to adhere to, as some infants are perceived to spit up less or are more easily

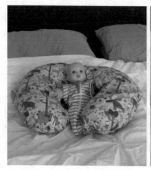 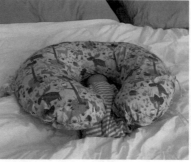

FIGURE 8.3 Hypothetical death scene based on death scene investigation. The left frame shows the infant was propped against a U-shaped pillow on a bed. Once asleep the infant slid off the pillow and fell to prone with the pillow coming over her head (right frame). (Permission Rebecca Carlin)

soothed on an incline. While regulations require inclined sleepers and positioners to carry suffocation risk warnings on them, and the product manual often explicitly states these products are not safe for sleep, they are often marketed for just that. It may be hard for families to understand the safety risk when the infant is strapped into a swing or other seating device and appears stable. Furthermore, the use of some of these products in hospitals is widespread, as they provide a place for the infant to be visible while nurses are caring for other patients. This modeling may result in parents presuming that these products are safe despite the product label advising against use for sleep. Since the CPSC report, many of these products have also been recalled, but as families often receive them as hand-me-downs or gifts, they may be unaware of the recall.

Counseling Families About Inclined Sleepers and Positioners

Given the often conflicting messaging that parents receive from marketers espousing the benefits of inclined sleepers or positioners, clear, consistent messaging about the safety risk associated with use of these products as infant sleep surfaces from the early newborn period is of utmost importance. This includes training nurses not to prop up one end of the bassinet in the nursery, as this remains a common practice. Encouraging parents to read the safety information in the product handbook or accessing it online to show parents while in the office can be effective to helping them understand the risk of the specific product they are using. Using images or demonstrating the instability of such positions in the office can also be helpful.

Parents also need an alternative plan in place for when infants become fussy or colicky. An infant who has been sleeping in an inclined swing is likely to cry for some period when placed flat on their back on a firm surface. Talking to families in advance about this likelihood and discussing other soothing techniques in advance (see Chap. 5) can empower parents in a stressful situation when it occurs. In instances where using such chairs or devices is required (e.g., during travel), the AAP specifically advises that if infants fall asleep in a sitting or inclined device, including a car seat, during travel, they should remain in the car seat until travel is completed. As soon as it is safe and practical, they can then be moved to a crib or other appropriate flat surface [18].

Crib Bumpers

Crib bumpers or other linings of crib slats were initially designed (prior to CPSC crib regulations [8]) to prevent head entrapment and subsequent strangulation. Reports of deaths associated with bumpers include cases of strangulation from the bumper ties, entrapment between bumper and mattress or crib side, and suffocation against bumper surfaces [19]. In response to the latter, some newer bumpers made of mesh and other breathable materials are being marketed as safe alternatives. While these alternative materials may decrease the risk of rebreathing, there are currently no standards defining the necessary permeability of such material, and the risk of strangulation is not decreased with altered material [19]. There is currently an international voluntary standard that all bumpers carry a suffocation warning as well as guidance to keep the straps tight and well secured [20]. Given the requirement for less than 2–3/8 inches between crib slats, there is no longer a risk of head entrapment in a crib, and the AAP specifically recommends that bumpers be avoided [18].

Common Barriers to Adherence

While the use of bumpers has decreased, parents who use them cite concern about entrapment, most commonly of limbs [9]. Despite the suffocation warning on them, marketing of newer breathable or mesh bumpers and vertical bumpers may convince parents that they are safe alternatives.

Counseling Parents

Although some parents may actively seek provider guidance on crib standards, the first step in counseling parents on a safe sleep environment is assuring that they know that the standards exist and are aware of what they are. For parents using used or older equipment that they believe may not meet the newest standards or have limited financial resources, low-cost programs for safe sleep spaces (e.g., cribs or play yards) are available in most regions (see Resources at end of book). Parents should be specifically advised that broken cribs should not be "repaired," as inadequate fixes can lead to unstable parts and potential injury.

With regard to bumpers, it is typically helpful to discuss the suffocation and strangulation risk that exists, even with products marked as "breathable." While there is the potential for an injured limb from entrapment in crib slats, these reports are uncommon and usually in children older than 6 months (note: safety warnings on bumpers caution that they are not to be used after an infant is 6 months of age), and the risks are far outweighed by bumper-related deaths [21].

Sheets and Loose Bedding

It is recommended that the only bedding in an infant sleep surface is a tightly fitted sheet. Loose bedding, including additional sheets, blankets, and stuffed animals, pose a risk of suffocation, should the bedding cover the infant's face (Figs. 8.4 and 8.5), and strangulation, should it get wrapped around the infant's neck. The AAP specifies that the sleep area should be clear of any strings, wires, or other objects that could wrap around the neck given cases of infants getting strangulated or hung from such objects.

Although it is safest if infants sleep without blankets, some have recommended that if a blanket is used, it should be thin, and the infant should be placed with the feet at the foot of the crib ("feet to foot"), with the blanket tucked in on three sides below the infant's armpits. However, although this advice makes sense to avoid infant head covering, there have been no studies to support that this is protective. Recently, use of an infant wearable blanket has been recommended by some safety advocates, including the AAP, as preferred over loose blankets. The wearable blanket should be the correct size for the infant, with a fitted neck and armholes or sleeves to keep the baby warm and no hood to avoid any chance of head covering or overheating. A case-control study in the Netherlands found that infants using cotton sleeping sacks (i.e., wearable blankets) were at lower risk for SIDS [22].

In the early newborn period, swaddling an infant is often recommended to help the infant settle to sleep in the supine position and keep blankets safely away from the face. Swaddled infants should always be placed supine to sleep, and swaddling should be stopped as soon as infants show any signs of being able to roll. Evidence for this comes from a meta-analysis that identified that swaddling risk varied

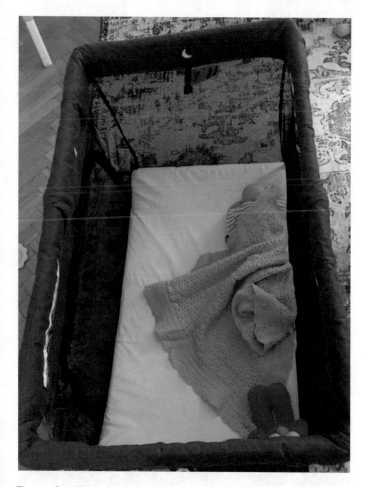

FIGURE 8.4 Hypothetical death scene in which infant was placed in play yard with blanket. The blanket came over her face as she rolled prone and was unable to recover. (Permission Rebecca Carlin)

according to position placed for sleep; the risk was highest for prone sleeping (OR, 12.99 [95% CI, 4.14–40.77]), followed by side sleeping (OR, 3.16 [95% CI, 2.08–4.81]), and supine sleeping (OR, 1.93 [95% CI, 1.27–2.93]) [23]. There

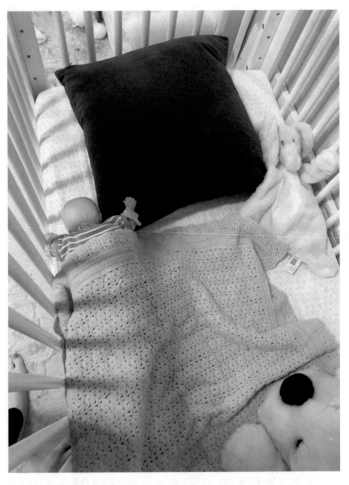

FIGURE 8.5 Hypothetical infant death scene based on death scene investigation in which the infant was placed in a crib with a pillow and soft bedding. The infant rolled to prone and was unable to recover. (Permission Rebecca Carlin)

was evidence to suggest swaddling risk increased with infant age and was associated with a two-fold risk for infants aged >6 months [23].

Common Barriers to Adherence

Parents using loose bedding are usually motivated by a desire to keeping infants warm. They may not know about, or own wearable alternatives to sheets or blankets. As infants get older, they may find comfort in holding a stuffed animal or other small blanket, and during sleep training, parents may be loathe to take the comfort object from the child at bedtime. Additionally, although the safe to sleep guidelines and hand-outs include warnings about soft bedding, parents are more aware of the recommendation for back to sleep and so may not appropriately recognize the risk to their infants. Finally, loose bedding is almost always present on shared sleep surfaces, making it hard to avoid for parents who wish to bed-share.

Counseling Families About Sheets and Loose Bedding

Parents who are using loose bedding often just need to be presented with the risk of strangulation and alternative options of wearable blankets. If parents are concerned that their child will be cold, layers of clothing should be recommended as an alternative to blankets. Particularly as children start to roll, families are more able to comprehend the theoretical risk of getting "stuck in the sheet or blanket." Using the terminology of suffocation or strangulation and explaining the mechanism is often helpful [6]. For those parents who are choosing to bed-share, it is important to review with them that the presence of loose bedding increases the dangers of that scenario.

If parents are using soft bedding as a soothing technique for an infant, it can be challenging to find an alternative. It is often necessary to discuss the risk and try to troubleshoot individual alternatives while also reviewing age-appropriate sleep training techniques. Having a conversation about loose bedding early in infancy before the association of a soft bedding comfort object and sleep has been established is particularly helpful in preventing this challenge.

Pillows

Pillows are the most common object involved in sleep-related infant deaths [2, 7]. As stated above, infants with pillows in their sleep environment have an almost three times higher risk of SIDS [1]. Similar to a soft mattress, a pillow can conform to the infant's head and can create an environment that may facilitate suffocation, particularly if she is in the prone position intentionally or accidentally (see Fig. 8.1). A plush pillow poses the potential additional hazard of covering an infant's airway, as a sheet or blanket might. Placing an infant's body completely or partially on top of a pillow adds the additional hazard of slipping off the pillow and becoming wedged under it or against another object, as can happen with a positioner (Fig. 8.5).

Common Barriers to Adherence

Common reasons for pillow use include the perception that the infant will be more comfortable lying on or with a pillow. Some parents may use the pillow to position a baby (e.g., on the side). Pillows are also often present in a shared sleep environment; sometimes this is because the parent is using the pillow for his or her own comfort. Some parents will also use the pillow as a barrier for the baby, so that the baby will not fall off the bed or that the parent will not roll into the baby.

Counseling Parents Against Pillow Use

The good thing about pillows is that unlike unsafe cribs or mattresses, there is no replacement necessary – they can just be removed! Discussing the safety hazard they pose and marked increased risk of SIDS is often enough to get them removed from an unshared sleep surface. Parents can be reassured that infants are comfortable sleeping flat without a pillow. When parents disclose that they are using a shared sleep surface, they should be told of the additional risks that pillows pose in that setting and be discouraged from using them if they continue to choose to bed-share.

Frequently Asked Questions

1. *Do children with gastroesophageal reflux benefit from being on an incline, either on an already inclined sleep surface or on a positioner?*

   No. There is no evidence that being on a partial incline reduces reflux symptoms, and most studies show the symptoms at a partial incline are similar to those on a flat sleep surface. Given the risk of sliding to the end of the inclined sleep surface or off of the positioner, all infants, including those with gastroesophageal reflux, should sleep on a flat surface. In fact, this risk was considered so significant that the CPSC recalled inclined sleepers in 2019 after reports of more than 30 deaths. Infants with GE reflux may benefit from being held fully upright by an adult after eating and then placed on a flat surface for sleep [24].

2. *Is it safe for my infant to sleep in an infant sling or carrier?*

   Infant slings and carriers are not the preferred sleep location for any infant. However, parents using these devices to carry the infant should position the baby safely, in case the baby falls asleep while being carried. The infant's head should always be up above the fabric with his face visible, and caregivers must ensure his nose and mouth are clear from obstructions. Infants who nurse while in a sling should be repositioned as above once feeding is completed.

3. *Can I use a crib my friend gave me? Would it be okay to replace the mattress it came with?*

It is preferable to use a new crib. However, you can use a used crib, provided it meets CPSC standards. Prior to use, you should ensure that the crib meets the current standard and has not been recalled. The crib should also be inspected for broken, missing, or loose parts, which may mean it does not meet safety standards. If the crib is damaged, you should not attempt to repair it, as inadequate repairs often lead to injury.

Crib mattresses can be replaced, provided that the replacement mattress is designated for the specific crib. In checking to ensure that the replacement is safe, make sure that it complies with standard firmness and thickness regulations and there is no gap between the mattress and the wall of the crib.

4. *Is it safe for me to have my baby on my bed if he is in a co-sleeper?*

In-bed co-sleepers are devices intended to give infants their own designated space on an adult bed. They are generally designed for use with two sober adults and young infants who cannot yet roll. There are many products on the market, ranging from a rectangular box with a firm bottom and mesh sides to devices with inflatable or cushioned sides. None of these devices have been rigorously evaluated for safety, and given the wide range of designs, it is difficult to make blanket statements about their safety. A 2015 review of CPSC reports regarding co-sleepers found 20 injuries and 6 deaths reported in co-sleepers. Five of the deaths were from asphyxia and one was from SIDS. Almost all of the infants had other risk factors for SIDS present, and half of all injuries and deaths occurred in co-sleepers that were improperly assembled [25].

Given that the safety of these devices has not been evaluated, the AAP did not make any recommendation for or against them in their 2016 safe sleep guidelines. While co-

sleepers appear to be associated with a relatively low incidence of injury and death, if parents opt to use them, they
should make sure that they are properly assembled; that they
are being used according to the manufacturer's guidelines in
terms of infant age, size, and developmental milestones; and
that the environment is free of other risk factors such as soft
bedding. Most, if not all, of these products carry a suffocation
warning for improper use, which parents should be alerted to.

Vignette Follow-Up

It is not uncommon for parents to position infants on pillows
and not disclose it unless specifically asked when talking
about the sleep environment. When counseling Avery's parents, it is important to understand why they placed her on a
U-shaped pillow. In this case, it was likely because she
sounded congested, but other parents may use similar positioners because of concerns about reflux or purely for comfort. When counseling parents, it is important to address these
concerns, whatever they may be, and to provide alternative
solutions or reassurance so that the parents feel empowered
to change the behavior. It is also important to discuss the
specific risks of soft bedding with Avery's parents. In this case,
you need to address both the U-shaped pillow and the loose
blanket. For the pillow, it is important to discuss the risk of
wedging and suffocation from the pillow itself as well as the
risk of falling off the pillow into the prone position. With
regard to the blanket, it could come over the infants face
leading to suffocation or wrap around the infants neck
leading to strangulation. Pictures or models made from common exam room items like top sheets can be utilized to
increase a family's understanding of potential hazards.

Clinical Pearls

1. The safest sleep environment for a baby is a firm, flat surface without anything around the infant.

2. Always counsel parents that when they are tired and concerned that there is a chance that they will fall asleep while feeding, the safest place to feed is in their bed without surrounding soft bedding. The risk of SUID is higher if they fall asleep on a couch or in a chair.
3. Understanding individual parental motivation for using soft bedding or soft sleep surfaces can be helpful in addressing concerns and fostering change.
4. When a provider is concerned about soft bedding use, using the word "suffocation" rather than SIDS or SUID may be helpful to get parents to understand the risks.
5. When purchasing infant products, parents should always read the warnings – many products are marketed as though they are safe for sleep but in fact have a warning that they are not a safe sleep surface.

References

1. Hauck FR, Herman SM, Donovan M, et al. Sleep environment and the risk of sudden infant death syndrome in an urban population: the Chicago Infant Mortality Study. Pediatrics. 2003;111:1207–14.
2. Erck Lambert AB, Parks SE, Cottengim C, Faulkner M, Hauck FR, Shapiro-Mendoza CK. Sleep-related infant suffocation deaths attributable to soft bedding, overlay, and wedging. Pediatrics. 2019;143:e20183408.
3. Moon RY. Task Force on Sudden Infant Death Syndrome, SIDS and other sleep-related infant deaths: updated 2016 recommendations for a safe infant sleeping environment. Pediatrics. 2016;138:e20162938.
4. Bombard JM, Kortsmit K, Warner L, et al. Vital signs: trends and disparities in infant safe sleep practices – United States, 2009–2015. MMWR Morb Mortal Wkly Rep. 2018;67:39–46.
5. Moon RY, Oden RP, Joyner BL, Ajao TI. Qualitative analysis of beliefs and perceptions about sudden infant death syndrome in African-American mothers: implications for safe sleep recommendations. J Pediatr. 2010;157:92–7.e2.

6. Mathews A, Joyner BL, Oden RP, He J, McCarter R Jr, Moon RY. Messaging affects the behavior of African American parents with regards to soft bedding in the infant sleep environment: a randomized controlled trial. J Pediatr. 2016;175:79–85.e2.

7. Gaw CE, Chounthirath T, Midgett J, Quinlan K, Smith GA. Types of objects in the sleep environment associated with infant suffocation and strangulation. Acad Pediatr. 2017;17:893–901.

8. U.S. Consumer Product Safety Commission, Office of Compliance, Requirements for Full Size Baby Cribs. Bethesda, MD; 2001.

9. Ajao TI, Oden RP, Joyner BL, Moon RY. Decisions of black parents about infant bedding and sleep surfaces: a qualitative study. Pediatrics. 2011;128:494–502.

10. Rechtman LR, Colvin JD, Blair PS, Moon RY. Sofas and infant mortality. Pediatrics. 2014;134:e1293–300.

11. Nelson SP, Chen EH, Syniar GM, Christoffel KK. Prevalence of symptoms of gastroesophageal reflux during infancy. A pediatric practice-based survey. Pediatric Practice Research Group. Arch Pediatr Adolesc Med. 1997;151:569–72.

12. Orenstein SR, Whitington PF, Orenstein DM. The infant seat as treatment for gastroesophageal reflux. N Engl J Med. 1983;309:760–3.

13. Mannen EM, Carroll J, Bumpass DB, et al. Biomechanical analysis of inclined sleep products. Little Rock: Univeristy of Arkansas; 2019.

14. Rosen R, Vandenplas Y, Singendonk M, et al. Pediatric gastroesophageal reflux clinical practice guidelines: joint recommendations of the North American Society for Pediatric Gastroenterology, Hepatology, and Nutrition and the European Society for Pediatric Gastroenterology, Hepatology, and Nutrition. J Pediatr Gastroenterol Nutr. 2018;66:516–54.

15. Commission CS. Supplemental notice of proposed rulemaking for infant sleep products.

16. Byard RW, Beal SM. V-shaped pillows and unsafe infant sleeping. J Paediatr Child Health. 1997;33:171–3.

17. Cottengim C, Parks SE, Erck Lambert AB, et al. U-shaped pillows and sleep-related infant deaths, United States, 2004–2015. Matern Child Health J 2020; 24, 222–8.

18. Moon RY, Task Force On Sudden Infant Death S. SIDS and other sleep-related infant deaths: evidence base for 2016

updated recommendations for a safe infant sleeping environment. Pediatrics. 2016;138: e20162940.

19. Scheers NJ, Woodard DW, Thach BT. Crib Bumpers Continue to Cause Infant Deaths: A Need for a New Preventive Approach. J Pediatr. 2016;169:93–7.e1.

20. ASTM International. F1917-20 Standard Consumer Safety Performance Specification for Infant Bedding and Related Accessories. West Conshohocken, PA, 2020. Web. 18 May 2020.

21. Yeh ES, Rochette LM, McKenzie LB, Smith GA. Injuries associated with cribs, playpens, and bassinets among young children in the US, 1990–2008. Pediatrics. 2011;127:479–86.

22. L'Hoir MP, Engelberts AC, van Well GTJ, et al. Risk and preventive factors for cot death in The Netherlands, a low-incidence country. Eur J Pediatr. 1998;157:681–8.

23. Pease AS, Fleming PJ, Hauck FR, et al. Swaddling and the risk of sudden infant death syndrome: a meta-analysis. Pediatrics. 2016;137

24. Lightdale JR, Gremse DA. Gastroesophageal reflux: management guidance for the pediatrician. Pediatrics. 2013;131:e1684–95.

25. Thompson EL, Moon RY. Hazard patterns associated with co-sleepers. Clin Pediatr (Phila). 2016;55:645–9.

Chapter 9
Baby Products: How to Evaluate Them for Potential Safety

Jeffrey D. Colvin

Clinical Vignette

You are seeing a healthy 1-month-old female in clinic for a well-child checkup. When you ask about sleep, the parents state that their daughter has difficulty sleeping. However, she sleeps much better now that she is swaddled and uses an in-bed sleeper. Before you can respond, the parents state that they feel the in-bed sleeper is safe because it keeps the infant on her back when sleeping. You have never heard any concerns about in-bed sleepers. Could it be a safe alternative to a crib, bassinet, or play yard?

"Bare Is Best"

With regard to an infant's sleep environment, the US Consumer Product Safety Commission (CPSC) gives the best advice: "bare is best," [1] meaning that the only baby products that should be in an infant's sleep environment are:

- Crib, bassinet, portable crib, or play yard.
- Firm crib mattress.

J. D. Colvin (✉)
Pediatrics, Children's Mercy Kansas City, Kansas City, MO, USA
e-mail: jdcolvin@cmh.edu

© Springer Nature Switzerland AG 2020
R. Y. Moon (ed.), *Infant Safe Sleep*,
https://doi.org/10.1007/978-3-030-47542-0_9

- Fitted sheet covering the mattress.
- Pacifier.

Everything else is a potential suffocation hazard, and parents should be instructed to remove them. Specifically, parents should be told that the following items do *not* benefit the infant, could create a suffocation risk, and should be removed:

- Bumper pads [2, 3].
- Any pillows (including breastfeeding pillows) [4–6].
- Stuffed animals.
- Positioners and wedges [7].
- Quilts [4, 5, 8].

Some products make claims of enhancing safe sleep but ultimately may pose more of a danger. For instance, positioners and wedges may claim to keep an infant in a specific position, including the supine position, during sleep. However, it is equally possible that such devices can be associated with suffocation (Fig. 9.1) [7].

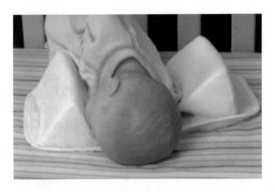

Figure 9.1 Example of suffocation in an infant positioner. (Source: https://www.cpsc.gov/Newsroom/Video/sleep-positioners-a-suffocation-risk)

Recommendations for a Safe Crib, Bassinet, or Play Yard: Buy It New!

Using a crib, bassinet, or play yard for sleep is key to infant safe sleep [9]. There is no evidence that supports one of these sleep areas over the others. By purchasing a new crib, bassinet, or play yard, parents can be more assured that the item meets current CPSC standards. Those standards were last updated in 2014 and include such safety features as the maximum slat spacing (no more than 2–3/8″), slat strength, and no drop sides [10].

Checking for Recalls

Before purchasing an item, parents can check the CPSC website for recalls of the item, as it may have been recalled but not removed by the seller. This can be easily done by going to the CPSC website (www.cpsc.gov) and entering the name of the product in the search box. This allows individuals to search for recalls on specific products. Once purchased, most cribs, bassinets, and play yards also have ways for purchasers to register the product with the manufacturer, either through a registration card or on the product's website. By registering the product, the purchasers will be informed of any recalls.

Periodic Inspections

Some products may be initially safe when purchased but become unsafe through deterioration of the product with use [6, 8]. As a result, the product should be inspected for its durability: Is it sturdy? Will it tip over? Does it appear to be well made? It should also be periodically inspected to ensure that it remains safe and not in need of repairs. Cribs, bassinets, and play yards that are broken, not correctly assembled, or which become disassembled due to loose screws or attachments can result in entrapment of the infant (Fig. 9.2) [6, 8, 11, 12].

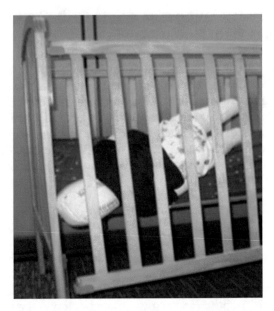

FIGURE 9.2 Entrapment due to broken crib. (Source: https://www.cpsc.gov/s3fs-public/simplicity.pdf)

Caution Against Using Used or Older Cribs

Older cribs may not meet current CPSC standards and are potentially dangerous. As a result, parents should be encouraged to purchase a new crib, bassinet, or play yard. Cribs, bassinets, and play yards older than 10 years should not be used. If cost is an issue, there are options to make purchasing a safe sleep area more affordable. (See Resources at end of book.) If obtaining a new crib, bassinet, or play yard is still not possible, the family should be instructed to examine the crib for the following dangerous features: [13].

- Drop sides (side of the crib slides down).
- Spaces between slats wider than 2 3/8″ (the width of a soda can).
- Broken or loose slats.

- Missing screws, brackets, or other hardware.
- Any holes/cutouts in the headboard or footboard.
- V-folding sides (portable cribs or play yards).
- Portable cribs or play yards with any damage to the mesh sides or mesh with spacing larger than ¼".
- Unstable legs that could result in the crib, bassinet, or play yard falling or tipping.
- Unstable frame allowing space between the mattress and the crib, bassinet, or play yard.

What Is Not a Crib, Bassinet, or Play Yard

Unfortunately, families will frequently use products that are not a crib, bassinet, or play yard for their infant's sleep. It may be that these items are perceived by parents as being safe since they are marketed for infants (e.g., swings) or they are specifically used for safety (e.g., car seats).

It can be difficult for parents to understand why certain products designed for infant safety (e.g., car seats) or that undergo CPSC approval are not also safe for sleep. The answer is a matter of *relative* safety: those products may be safe while the infant is awake or may be safest location when the infant is travelling in a vehicle but are not as safe when the infant is sleeping and not in a vehicle. Between 2004 and 2014, there were 348 infant sleep-related deaths in sitting devices, including car seats and swings [14]. More than 90% of these deaths occurred while the device was not being used as recommended (e.g., the device was being used at home, or the infant was not appropriately strapped in). The elements of those products that improve their safety, such as padding, straps, and an inclined sitting angle, make them more dangerous when the infant is asleep and not travelling. Consequently, if an infant falls asleep in a car seat, swing, or other sitting device, he should be removed from the car seat as the destination is reached or removed from the swing or other sitting device and placed in a bassinet, crib, or play yard as soon as it is safe to do so.

A Safe Crib Mattress Is a *Hard, Tightly Fitting* Crib Mattress

Like cribs, bassinets, portable cribs, and play yards, crib mattresses should also ideally be purchased new in order to assure that they meet current CPSC requirements [15, 16]. This will ensure that the mattress meets specific standards regarding flammable materials, thickness, and firmness. Recalls of specific mattresses can be checked in the same way that recalls of other products are checked.

When purchasing a crib mattress, there are two critical characteristics that parents should look for:

1. *A Tight Fit.* Each crib should state the appropriate size of mattress for that model. The mattress should fit tightly within the crib structure. Parents can best assure this by making sure the mattress dimensions are the same as the crib. If this is true, it should take some force to set the mattress on its base inside the crib. This means there should be no gaps between the mattress and the sides of the crib frame, and it should be tight when inserting a hand between a side of the crib frame and the mattress. There should never be more than a width of two fingers between the mattress and the crib [1].
2. *The Mattress Should Be Hard.* Although crib mattresses should be "firm," in practical terms, it should feel *hard* to an adult. It should not feel like an adult mattress. As a result, the mattress *should not indent* when an infant is lying on it. Parents often misunderstand what "firm" means, and additional specification is needed [17]. Why is a hard mattress required? It is required because any soft object in the sleep environment can potentially indent, thereby occluding an infant's nose and mouth and result in suffocation (Fig. 9.3).

Fitted Crib Mattress Sheets

A "fitted" mattress sheet is one with elastic sewn into the corners so that it wraps around the mattress corners. Unfortunately, if an appropriate fitted crib sheet is not

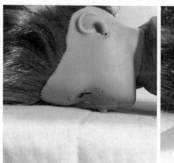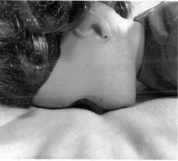

Firm mattress   Soft mattress

FIGURE 9.3 Crib mattresses should *not* indent when an infant lies on them

purchased or properly used, the sheet can become a suffocation hazard. In selecting a fitted crib mattress sheet, parents should look for the following: [18].

- Do not use an adult sheet or crib sheet that is not "fitted."
- The fitted crib sheet should be for the specific dimensions of the crib mattress.
- The fitted sheet should wrap completely around all four sides of the mattress so that sheet ends on the bottom of the mattress. This helps the fitted sheet stay in place. The tight fit between the sides of the crib and the mattress should also help keep the sheet in place.
- The fitted sheet should fit tightly on the mattress. There should be minimal to no slack in the sheet when on the mattress.
- It should be *very* difficult to remove the sheet without removing the mattress from the crib.
- The infant should never sleep on top of other bedding, including mattress toppers, blankets, sheepskin blankets, quilts, comforters, and pillows.

Top Sheets, Swaddle Sacks, and Other Bedding

Top sheets are the linens that cover one's body during sleep. Due to the potential for suffocation or strangulation, the AAP now recommends that *no* sheets or blankets be used [9].

Swaddling and swaddle sacks are linens that wrap around an infant's body to provide warmth or comfort. The research is mixed on whether swaddling is a risk or protective factor for sleep-related infant deaths. A recent review of the four studies on swaddling was unable to make any definitive conclusions about all swaddling and the risk of SIDS [19]. However, it did find a very high risk of death in swaddled infants >6 months old and when the combination of swaddling and the prone or side sleep positions was used. Like all products in the sleep environment, swaddling blankets are a potential suffocation risk if they become loose. Although swaddle sacks do not have some of the risks inherent in swaddling with a blanket, there are no studies assessing their safety. The AAP's most recent guidelines do not recommend for or against swaddling or swaddle sacks [9].

When counseling families on swaddling and the use of swaddle sacks, the following recommendations can be made: [20].

- When the infant reaches the age that he or she is trying to roll (i.e., usually 2–4 months of age), swaddling should no longer be used.
- Babies should be placed only on their backs when swaddled.
- *Tight* swaddling is associated with worsening of other health conditions, such as restricted breathing or hip dysplasia, but *loose* swaddling can result in the blanket becoming free, thereby becoming a suffocation risk.
- Swaddle sacks should be of an appropriate size for the infant so that the infant's head does not slip into sack, which can lead to suffocation.

- Avoid overheating: over swaddling an infant can cause overheating, which is a risk factor for SIDS.
- One alternative to swaddling or swaddle sacks, especially if warmth is the primary concern, is for the infant to wear a second infant sleeper when sleeping. As with swaddling, the parent should ensure that overheating does not occur.
- Other than swaddling with a light blanket or using a swaddle sack, no other bedding should be used, including other blankets, sheepskin blankets, quilts, comforters, and pillows [4, 5, 8, 21].

Bedside and In-Bed Co-Sleepers

Bedside and in-bed co-sleepers are newer products marketed for infant sleep. They are bassinet-like sleep areas than either attach to the parents' bed ("bedside") or are designed to be placed in the parents' bed. The CPSC currently has safety standards for bedside co-sleepers [22]. Bedside co-sleepers allow parents to have arms-reach access to their infant (in a manner similar to bed-sharing), while allowing their infant to have a separate sleep space. There are no similar safety standards for in-bed co-sleepers. There is concern that some products marketed as co-sleepers have soft padded sides or surfaces that may create risk.

While no studies on commercially produced bedside or in-bed co-sleepers have been published, there has been one small (n-200) randomized controlled trial of a traditional, flax-woven in-bed sleeper (wahakura) specific to the indigenous population of New Zealand. When compared to babies randomized to sleep in a bassinet, babies in the wahakura had similar oxygen saturation, mean heart rate, and body temperature, and babies sleeping in the wahakura had higher breastfeeding rates [23]. Although increased use of wahakuras (and a similar product called a pēpi-pod) in recent years has been associated with fewer sleep-related infant deaths in New Zealand, it is unclear if it is the device, the accompanying widespread safe sleep education efforts, or other factors that have contributed to the reductions in mortality [24].

Baby Monitors

Whether it's a monitor marketed to reduce SIDS or a more typical "baby monitor" which provides visual or audio communication to parents, there's one thing to remember: several research studies, conducted with hospital-grade monitors, have demonstrated that none of these monitors will prevent a sleep-related infant death [25–27]. Further, current commercially available baby monitors may have electrical cords and other possible items that could create a strangulation risk. Newer monitoring devices that are wearable like a sock and which can provide data on the infant's heart rate and oxygen saturation to the parent's smart phone have been developed. However, these devices performed very poorly and were determined to be unreliable when tested against hospital-grade monitors [28]. This does not mean that monitors should never be used. There are specific indications unrelated to SIDS in which a physician may prescribe a medical monitor (e.g., pulse oximeter for an infant with chronic hypoxia due to chronic lung disease or a Holter monitor for an infant with a suspected arrhythmia).

However, there are concerns that monitor use will lead to parental complacency about following safe sleep guidelines. Use of even the most high-tech monitor should not replace safe sleep behaviors.

Assessing New Products

There are multiple other products marketed for infant sleep. Some of them are marketed for the prevention of SIDS. For all of these products, providers counseling parents should remember "buyer beware!" and the following principles:

- The CPSC has warned against the use of any inclined infant sleeping device [29]. (See Chap. 8 for a more detailed discussion of inclined sleeping devices.)
- Just because it is marketed for infants and sold in a well-respected store or website does not make it safe.
- There is no routine safety testing that is required before products are sold. The only products that are regulated by the FDA are devices that make a medical claim (e.g., to prevent suffocation or to relieve gastroesophageal reflux). For most products, there are no CPSC standards.
- Just because a product has met CPSC standards does not make it safe. CPSC standards regulate against obvious hazards, but CPSC only removes a product from the market after several deaths have been reported.
- Some of these products have features such as an inclined or soft sleep surface or padding that makes them unsafe.
- Without further research to the contrary, it must be presumed that these products cannot make an unsafe sleep environment safe (e.g., bed-sharing with an in-bed sleeper) – two wrongs do not make a right.
- If the product claims to allow you to not follow safe sleep guidelines without risk, it is likely not safe.
- The safest place for an infant to sleep is in a bare crib, bassinet, or play yard.

Frequently Asked Questions

How can a family determine if a used crib is safe?

It is best to buy a new crib, bassinet or play yard. However, sometimes that is not possible. The family should check to make sure that the crib meets CPSC standards and has not been recalled. Cribs, bassinets, and play yards that are more than 10 years old should not be used (they will not meet CPSC standards). The crib should also be inspected for broken, missing, or loose parts, which may mean it does not meet safety standards. If the crib is damaged, the family should not attempt to repair it, as inadequate repairs often lead to injury.

Crib mattresses can be replaced, provided that the replacement mattress is designated for the specific crib. In checking to ensure that the replacement is safe, make sure that it complies with standard firmness and thickness regulations and there is no gap between the mattress and the wall of the crib.

Are portable cribs and play yards as safe as cribs and bassinets?

Although there is no research comparing portable cribs and play yards to cribs and bassinets, it is believed that they are equally safe so long as the portable crib or play yard is new, meets CPSC standards, and is in good condition.

Are car seats and infant swings acceptable alternatives to cribs, bassinets, and play yards?

No, infant swings, car seats, and other sitting devices are not acceptable alternatives. If an infant falls asleep in a car seat, swing, or other infant seat, she should be moved to a crib, bassinet, or play yard, unless the infant is in a car seat and actively in transit.

Is swaddling safe? Do swaddle sacks reduce the risk of a sleep-related death?

We do not know. The research is mixed on swaddling and there is no research on swaddle sacks. When an infant begins to show signs of rolling over, the infant should no longer be swaddled. Swaddled babies should only be supine. It is also important to ensure that the swaddle sack fits the infant correctly and that the material used for swaddling cannot cause suffocation or strangulation.

Are there any monitors that reduce the risk of SIDS?

No. Prescribed medical monitors should only be used for previously diagnosed or suspected conditions (e.g., a pulse oximeter for hypoxia secondary to chronic lung disease).

Are bedside sleepers or in-bed sleepers safe?

We do not know. There is no current research comparing the safety of bedside sleepers and in-bed sleepers to cribs, bassinets, and play yards. As a result, current guidelines continue to recommend cribs, bassinets, and play yards.

What if I have a problem with a baby product or am worried that it is dangerous?

You can report incidents or accidents (even near-accidents) to the Consumer Product Safety Commission at https://www.saferproducts.gov/CPSRMSPublic/Incidents/ReportIncident.aspx

Vignette Follow-Up

You respond by first praising the patient's parents for wanting their infant to sleep on her back. You also empathize with their struggle to improve their infant's sleep. You explain that there are few data on whether in-bed co-sleepers are safe and that they are not tested or regulated by the CPSC. The parents were surprised to hear that the government did not first test a product sold for infants. You discuss alternatives, including those that are provided at no cost by nonprofit organizations.

Clinical Pearls

- The safest place for an infant to sleep is in a crib, basinet, portable crib, or play yard.
- New is best for cribs, bassinets, play yards, and mattresses.
- Crib mattresses should be "firm" (i.e., hard). The mattress should *not* indent when the infant is laying on it. The mattress should also fit snugly against the crib on all four sides.
- The only other object in the crib, bassinet, or play yard should be a fitted sheet, which should fit snugly on the mattress and wrap around to the bottom of the mattress on all four sides.
- Just because a product is marketed for infants and sold in a well-respected store or website does not make it safe.
- If the product claims to allow you to not follow safe sleep guidelines without risk, it is likely not safe.

References

1. United States Consumer Product Safety Commission. Safe sleep – cribs and infant products information center. https://www.cpsc.gov/SafeSleep. Accessed February 2, 2020.
2. Scheers NJ, Woodard DW, Thach BT. Crib bumpers continue to cause infant deaths: a need for a new preventive approach. J Pediatr. 2016;169:93–7.e91.
3. Thach BT, Rutherford GW, Jr, Harris K. Deaths and injuries attributed to infant crib bumper pads. J Pediatr. 2007;151(3):271–4, 274.e271–273.
4. Gaw CE, Chounthirath T, Midgett J, Quinlan K, Smith GA. Types of objects in the sleep environment associated with infant suffocation and strangulation. Acad Pediatr. 2017;17(8):893–901.
5. Scheers NJ, Dayton CM, Kemp JS. Sudden infant death with external airways covered: case-comparison study of 206 deaths in the United States. Arch Pediatr Adolesc Med. 1998;152(6):540–7.
6. Drago DA, Dannenberg AL. Infant mechanical suffocation deaths in the United States, 1980–1997. Pediatrics. 1999;103(5):e59.
7. Suffocation deaths associated with use of infant sleep positioners–United States, 1997–2011. MMWR Morb Mortal Wkly Rep. 2012;61(46):933–7.
8. Li L, Fowler D, Liu L, Ripple MG, Lambros Z, Smialek JE. Investigation of sudden infant deaths in the State of Maryland (1990-2000). Forensic Sci Int. 2005;148(2–3):85–92.
9. SIDS and other sleep-related infant deaths: updated 2016 recommendations for a safe infant sleeping environment. Pediatrics 2016;138(5):1–12.
10. United States Consumer Product Safety Commission. Full-size cribs. https://www.cpsc.gov/Regulations-Laws%2D%2DStandards/Rulemaking/Final-and-Proposed-Rules/Full-Size-Cribs. Accessed February 2, 2020.
11. Hayman RM, McDonald G, Baker NJ, Mitchell EA, Dalziel SR. Infant suffocation in place of sleep: New Zealand national data 2002–2009. Arch Dis Child. 2015;100(7):610–4.
12. Jackson A, Moon RY. An analysis of deaths in portable cribs and playpens: what can be learned? Clin Pediatr. 2008;47(3):261–6.
13. United States Consumer Product Safety Commission. Crib safety Tips. https://www.cpsc.gov/safety-education/safety-guides/cribs/crib-safety-tips. Accessed February 2, 2020.

14. Liaw P, Moon RY, Han A, Colvin JD. Infant deaths in sitting devices. Pediatrics. 2019;144:(1)1–7.
15. Brooke H, Gibson A, Tappin D, Brown H. Case-control study of sudden infant death syndrome in Scotland, 1992–5. BMJ (Clinical Research ed). 1997;314(7093):1516–20.
16. Tappin D, Brooke H, Ecob R, Gibson A. Used infant mattresses and sudden infant death syndrome in Scotland: case-control study. BMJ (Clinical Research ed). 2002;325(7371):1007.
17. Ajao TI, Oden RP, Joyner BL, Moon RY. Decisions of black parents about infant bedding and sleep surfaces: a qualitative study. Pediatrics. 2011;128(3):494–502.
18. United States Consumer Product Safety Commission. CPSC safety alert: crib sheets. https://www.cpsc.gov/s3fs-public/5137.pdf. Accessed February 2, 2020.
19. Pease AS, Fleming PJ, Hauck FR, et al. Swaddling and the risk of sudden infant death syndrome: a meta-analysis. Pediatrics. 2016;137(6):1–9.
20. Moon RY. SIDS and other sleep-related infant deaths: evidence base for 2016 updated recommendations for a safe infant sleeping environment. Pediatrics 2016;138(5):e1–e34.
21. Mitchell EA, Thompson JM, Ford RP, Taylor BJ. Sheepskin bedding and the sudden infant death syndrome. New Zealand Cot Death Study Group. J Pediatr. 1998;133(5):701–4.
22. Safety Standards for Bedside Sleepers. Federal Register 79: 2581 (2014).
23. Tipene-Leach D, Baddock SA, Williams SM, et al. The Pepi-Pod study: overnight video, oximetry and thermal environment while using an in-bed sleep device for sudden unexpected death in infancy prevention. J Paediatr Child Health. 2018;54(6):638–46.
24. Tipene-Leach D, Abel S. Innovation to prevent sudden infant death: the wahakura as an indigenous vision for a safe sleep environment. Aust J Prim Health. 2019;25(5):406–9.
25. Monod N, Plouin P, Sternberg B, et al. Are polygraphic and cardiopneumographic respiratory patterns useful tools for predicting the risk for sudden infant death syndrome? A 10-year study. Biol Neonate. 1986;50(3):147–53.
26. Ramanathan R, Corwin MJ, Hunt CE, et al. Cardiorespiratory events recorded on home monitors: comparison of healthy infants with those at increased risk for SIDS. JAMA. 2001;285(17):2199–207.

27. Ward SL, Keens TG, Chan LS, et al. Sudden infant death syndrome in infants evaluated by apnea programs in California. Pediatrics. 1986;77(4):451–8.
28. Bonafide CP, Localio AR, Ferro DF, et al. Accuracy of pulse oximetry-based home baby monitors. JAMA. 2018;320(7):717–9.
29. United States Consumer Product Safety Commission. CPSC cautions consumers not to use inclined infant sleep products. https://www.cpsc.gov/content/cpsc-cautions-consumers-not-to-use-inclined-infant-sleep-products. Accessed February 2, 2020.

Chapter 10
Special Situations: Co-occurring Health Conditions

Michael Goodstein

Clinical Vignette

Linda has brought her newborn daughter, Starr, into the office for their first visit since discharge from the neonatal intensive care unit 2 days ago. Linda has brought her mother along for support. The family has a lot of questions regarding the care of their baby, especially about safe sleep. Although this is Linda's second child, it is the first one she is directly caring for. Starr's older sibling, Johnny, is in foster care because Linda was using heroin during her first pregnancy. Linda is extremely bright and athletic but became addicted to pain killers after surgery for a career-ending college soccer injury. Unable to support her habit on the street, she turned to less expensive heroin to control her addiction. She is now stable in recovery on methadone, 85 mg daily and is hoping to attend college classes again part time.

Starr was born by Cesarean delivery at 34 weeks' gestation secondary to maternal preeclampsia and spent 26 days in the NICU. She had head-sparing intrauterine growth restriction with a birth weight of 1752 gms. Her hospital course was complicated by respiratory distress diagnosed as transient tachypnea of the newborn and she had moderate apnea of

M. Goodstein (✉)
Pediatrics, WellSpan York Hospital, York, PA, USA
e-mail: mgoodstein@wellspan.org

© Springer Nature Switzerland AG 2020
R. Y. Moon (ed.), *Infant Safe Sleep*,
https://doi.org/10.1007/978-3-030-47542-0_10

prematurity, requiring high flow nasal cannula for 1 week. Because of the respiratory support, Starr initially required gavage feedings. The hospital course was also complicated by neonatal abstinence syndrome (NAS). However, with Linda's commitment to rooming-in and providing extensive skin-to-skin care (SSC), Starr was able to avoid treatment with narcotic therapy.

Despite escaping the use of medication, Starr has been a fussy baby, and she has particularly struggled with feeding and weight gain. Linda notes that once Starr was well enough to nipple feed, it was difficult getting her to latch onto the breast despite working closely with the lactation counselors. The baby eventually required a feeding team assessment, as she had problems with both breast and bottle feedings. Starr also struggled with frequent regurgitation and poor weight gain. She was diagnosed with gastroesophageal reflux disease and was started on omeprazole, which she is still taking. Linda is worried that Starr is not growing despite being given supplements in the breast milk to increase its calories. Linda's mother comments that it would just be easier to give the baby formula, but Linda quickly scolds her, stating that her breast milk is healthier for Starr and can even reduce the risk of sudden infant death syndrome (SIDS). How do you counsel Starr's mother and grandmother?

The purpose of this chapter will be to review special situations that impact infant sleep safety and how to discuss overcoming potential barriers and resistance from families regarding these issues.

Gastroesophageal Reflux (GER)

Gastroesophageal reflux is an extremely common issue for infants and a big concern for new parents. It is critical that we help parents understand the difference between gastroesophageal reflux (GER) and gastroesophageal reflux disease (GERD). GER is an expected, naturally occurring phenomenon in newborns and is explained by a confluence of factors.

Compared to adult anatomy, the angle of His, or the gastro-esophageal junction is straighter, making it easier for gastric contents to reflux. As the angle of the junction increases with age, it becomes more difficult for reflux to occur. The infant anatomy also differs in having a relatively shorter esophagus and small stomach. Approximately 85% of infants vomit during the first week of life, and 60–70% manifest clinical gastro-esophageal reflux at age 3–4 months [1].

Normally, the lower esophageal sphincter (LES) relaxes during swallowing and during the passage of food down the esophagus. When swallowing is complete, the LES then contracts to maintain a higher pressure than the intragastric pressure to prevent reflux. Sudden transient relaxations of the lower esophageal sphincter (TLESRs), which are abrupt reflex decreases in LES pressure, unrelated to swallowing, to levels at or below intragastric pressure [2], allow the gastric contents to wash back into the esophagus when under the pressure of a full/distended stomach or during abdominal straining. To prevent regurgitation, esophageal contractions, including primary peristalsis and secondary contractions, usually terminate the TLESR and promote fast esophageal emptying of refluxate into the stomach [3]. Additionally, increased upper esophageal pressure and decreased relaxations may protect the larynx, pharynx, and lung from the harmful refluxate [4]. Maturation of the lower esophageal sphincter with increasing muscle tone also leads to dissipation of reflux events over the first year of life [5].

In the infant receiving human milk, there may be immune benefits from GER. Human milk contains immunoglobulins, lactoferrin, lysozyme, and white blood cells that are likely protective for infants. Antibodies in breast milk are reflective of the mother's GI and respiratory flora; infants have similar flora to their mothers, with maternal antibodies in the breast milk tailored for optimal protection (enteromammary immune system) [6]. Reflux allows these bioactive factors to stimulate the mucosal surfaces to prime the mucosa-associated lymphoid tissue and establish the commensal microbiome.

GER vs GERD

Parents need to be aware of the difference between GER (which is more of a nuisance issue) and GERD, which is a pathologic condition defined as GER that results in harm to the infant. The hallmark characteristics of GERD can include poor weight gain/failure to thrive and aspiration/pneumonia. Additionally, infants may develop esophagitis secondary to GERD, which may manifest by crying during feeding, refusal to eat, and/or arching after the feeding. However, the diagnosis can be challenging as many infants are irritable and cry frequently. It can be difficult to know whether the symptoms are a result of GERD.

Treatment Options for GERD

There are a handful of effective options for the appropriate treatment of GERD, according to the North American Society for Pediatric Gastroenterology, Hepatology, and Nutrition (NASPGAHN) and the European Society for Pediatric Gastroenterology, Hepatology, and Nutrition (ESPGAHN).

Feeding Modifications

Infants with GERD benefit from small, frequent feedings, whether breast or bottle feeding. Larger feeds can overdistend the stomach and promote reflux. Smaller feeds can also be beneficial if there is delayed gastric emptying. Additionally, if not breastfeeding, the formula can be thickened with rice or oatmeal cereal. Increasing viscosity will slow down the movement of the feeding and increase the force needed for reflux to occur. There are concerns regarding rice cereal and arsenic exposure. However, other grains may not dissolve as well and may cause clogging of the nipple.

Pros and Cons of Positioning as a Treatment for GERD

Keeping the baby in an upright position for 20–30 minutes after the feeding can help with GERD through the force of gravity [7]. Studies have suggested less reflux when the infant is in the prone position compared to supine [8, 9]. Therefore, it is acceptable to place an *awake* infant prone after a feeding if the baby is continuously monitored.

Although gastric emptying may be improved by placing the infant in the right side position, a handful of studies have shown a decrease in the number of TLESR-related reflux events when premature babies are placed in the left side position after feeding [9–11]. However, both prone and side positioning are associated with a two-fold increase in the risk of SIDS and are not recommended for the treatment of GERD in infants being placed for sleep.

Whereas keeping the baby upright after a feeding can help reduce GER, *it is not beneficial and can be potentially dangerous to place infants in an inclined position for sleep. Sitting devices (e.g., car seats) can place an infant in a position that increases pressure on the abdominal contents, which can exacerbate GER* [12]. There are additional concerns regarding airway obstruction and hypoxemia that can occur when the infant is on an inclined surface or in a sitting position if the head should tilt forward due to a lack of head control. Additionally, sitting devices, in particular, car seats, have soft materials that can create a suffocation hazard and straps that can lead to entanglement and suffocation. Even propping the mattress or using a home-made wedge can be hazardous, as these allow infants to roll down the crib and end up trapped in a non-supine position.

The FDA had approved several devices in the 1980s to help infants with GERD or with positional plagiocephaly. However, after a number of deaths reported to the CPSC, the FDA and CPSC, supported by the AAP, recommended that the devices no longer be produced or sold [13]. The FDA required that products claiming any medical benefit would need to be regulated by the FDA as medical devices and that manufacturers would have to demonstrate that the product benefit outweighed the risk of suffocation [13]. Many manufacturers dropped their claims of medical benefit, and thus many of these devices continue to be sold by retailers directly to the public as non-medical grade devices.

In 2019, inclined sleepers (which are frequently advertised as being beneficial for infants with reflux) came under additional scrutiny after a series of deaths were reported to the CPSC and additional deaths were uncovered in a Consumer Reports article [14]. Major manufacturers have voluntarily recalled their products, including 4.7 million units of the Fisher Price Rock N Play sleeper. The CPSC issued a statement for a supplemental proposed rule (Supplemental NPR), proposing to adopt the current ASTM standard for inclined sleep products, with modifications that would make the mandatory standard more stringent than the voluntary standard [15]. The proposed changes include limiting the seat back angle for sleep to 10 degrees or less.

Eliminating Tobacco Smoke

Eliminating tobacco smoke from the environment can also reduce GER. Studies in adults have demonstrated that tobacco smoke increases the frequency of GER events and prolongs esophageal acid clearance [16, 17]. Furthermore, discontinuation of tobacco smoke results in less severe GERD symptoms. In infants, perinatal smoke exposure has been linked to increased frequency of GER; in addition, when infants who have had prenatal smoke exposure do have GER, the regurgitant moves higher up the esophagus [18]. Smoking cessation will also provide the added benefit of reducing the risk of SUID.

Other Treatment Options

If GERD symptoms persist despite the above interventions, then a trial (2–4 weeks) of a protein hydrolysate or amino acid-based formula may be attempted. In one review, the authors found up to 15 to 40% of infants with GER(D) had a cow's milk protein intolerance or "dietary protein-induced gastroenteropathy." [19] In the case of breastfed infants, having the mother eliminate milk/dairy from her diet may be useful. Finally, if all else has failed, a trial of acid suppression therapy (4–8 weeks) may be indicated if the child cannot be evaluated by a pediatric gastroenterologist.

Guidance for Parents of an Infant with GER/ GERD

Anticipatory guidance should be directed by whether the baby has GER or GERD and the level of family anxiety. The baby with simple GER is often referred to as "the happy spitter." This infant regurgitates frequently but is in no discomfort and is growing well. Parents can be reassured that this is more of a messy/laundry issue than a health issue and is something the baby will outgrow. However, if the parents are very anxious, then sharing the basic interventions of more frequent, smaller feedings and keeping the baby upright after feedings may allay symptoms and parental concerns. Approximately 80% of infants will show improvement in their symptoms with this strategy.

For the infant who has actual GERD, it will be necessary to work through the progression of interventions previously discussed, starting with the environmental changes (positioning, small volume feeds), then changes in feeding (maternal diet if breastfeeding, elemental formula, thickened feeds) and finally acid-suppression therapy or pediatric gastroenterology consultation.

Regardless of whether the baby in question has GER or GERD, it will be critical to provide education regarding infant positioning when discussing therapeutic interventions with the family. Both the AAP Task Force on SIDS and NASPGAHN agree that *babies should be placed in the supine position for sleep regardless of the diagnosis of GER(D)*. The only exception would involve certain upper airway disorders for which the risk of death from reflux outweighs the risk of death from SUID. These are rare scenarios, such as grade 3 or 4 laryngeal cleft prior to surgical intervention.

Perhaps the biggest concern on the part of families is that the baby will choke or aspirate if they spit up while lying on the back. It is common for parents to mistake coughing and gagging for aspiration and a "life-threatening" event. They need reassurance that these sounds, although scary, are part of a normal, very powerful protective reflex that expels any liquid or material that tries to enter the airway. This is no different than what happens to us as adults when a bit of a drink "goes down the wrong pipe" and the resultant coughing fit, although unpleasant, can be embarrassing if one is out at the movies.

This author finds that one of the most helpful instruments for educating families (and healthcare providers) is an anatomic illustration (see Chap. 5, Fig. 5.1) showing the esophageal and tracheal anatomy in cross section in both the supine and prone positions. Showing parents that when gravity pushes regurgitation fluid to the lowest point in the back of the throat, they can see that it will pool around the airway more readily when the infant is in the prone position, increasing the risk of aspiration. In the supine position, the regurgitant will pool toward the esophagus, where it can be safely swallowed. This is also a good time to remind parents that neurologically intact infants will use their protective airway reflexes to cough up any liquid that enters the trachea.

Some families may be reassured by the data regarding back sleeping and aspiration. In the United States, the Back to Sleep® campaign led to a 52% reduction in SIDS over 10 years with no increase in the number of infants diagnosed with or dying of aspiration [20, 21]. These findings are consistent with those seen in other industrialized countries [22, 23].

Recent studies regarding parental choices of infant sleep behaviors suggest that subjective norms play a significant role in infant sleep and location [24, 25]. Providers can use this knowledge in discussions with families when exploring barriers to infant sleep safety. After acknowledging their concerns and providing the education outlined above, let them know back sleeping is the national norm in the United States and other industrialized countries. Approximately 75% of Americans routinely place their babies on the back for sleep [25, 26]. And one could conclude with noting that almost all of our patients chose back sleeping after having this discussion on the risks and benefits of different infant sleep positions.

Nasogastric (NG) Tubes

Although uncommon, there are instances when infants are discharged from the hospital with temporary NG feedings. Often the infants are premature: stable preterm infants may not have developed neurobehavioral maturity to nipple feed, while babies of extremely low birth weight may not have the stamina or respiratory stability secondary to chronic lung disease. Other infants will have tube feedings due to neurologic issues, such as perinatal asphyxia and subsequent hypoxic-ischemic encephalopathy or hypotonia and poor suck secondary to genetic disorders such as Prader-Willi syndrome.

There is concern that the use of an NG tube could worsen GER. One study of infants demonstrated an almost doubling of reflux events with an NG tube as opposed to one in the esophagus [27], and a second study found the risk for GERD increased with the length of time an NG tube is used in premature infants with bronchopulmonary dysplasia (BPD) [28]. It has been proposed that the mechanism of action is the NG tube causing a disruption of the lower esophageal sphincter function. However, a more recent 2018 study demonstrated that the presence of a 5-French NG tube was not associated with an increase in GER or acid exposure in preterm infants, and that infants fed through an NG tube actually had fewer episodes of GER [29].

Regardless of the uncertainty regarding any relationship between NG tubes and GER, there is no evidence that infants receiving NG or orogastric feedings are at increased risk of aspiration if placed in the supine position [21]. Parents should be given reassurance that back sleeping is the safest position for their baby, given that the leading cause of post-neonatal mortality is SUID and that the risk of death doubles when babies sleep on the stomach or side.

Hypothermia

Temperature regulation of the newborn is critical in the transition from the fetal life to the extrauterine environment. Newborns are at greater risk of hypothermia due to their larger body surface to mass ratio and limited subcutaneous tissue. There are multiple factors, including radiant heat, conduction, convection, and evaporation, which can lead to heat loss in infants. Newborns can transiently generate heat through brown fat stores (chemical non-shivering thermogenesis) found in the nape of the neck, the back, and around the kidneys [30].

Prevention of hypothermia at birth is important because studies have shown increased morbidity and mortality in preterm infants admitted to the intensive care nursery with low temperature [31, 32]. Thermal stress can be mitigated in the delivery room by good preparation prior to delivery with appropriate room temperature, warm blankets, and a radiant warmer [33]. The World Health Organization (WHO) recommends the delivery room temperature be at least 25–28 ° C (77.0–82.4 ° F) [34].

For the newly delivered healthy term infant, best practice is the immediate initiation of skin-to-skin care. Skin-to-skin care or kangaroo care has been shown to stabilize the newborn's temperature and help reduce the risk of hypothermia [35, 36]. The infants at greatest risk of hypothermia who are not already in the neonatal intensive care unit (NICU) are the late preterm infant, the low birth weight infant and the infant with intrauterine growth restriction/small for gestational age.

It is important for the clinical team in the hospital to model safe sleep while ensuring that the infant becomes neither hypothermic or overheated. Studies have shown that parents will make decisions about the home sleep environment based on what they see and how they are educated in the hospital [37–40]. Parents should be educated on how to keep their infants euthermic. The AAP Task Force on SIDS does not recommend a specific temperature range for the home environment, but instead recommends that *the room temperature be comfortable for a lightly dressed adult. The infant should be dressed in one additional layer of clothing. If the infant is having difficulty maintaining temperature, then additional layers of clothing should be added*. If a blanket is desired, it is preferable to use a wearable blanket rather than a receiving blanket or quilt. Wrapping or swaddling with blankets can pose many potential complications from increased respiratory rates to exacerbation of developmental hip dysplasia [21].

Blankets or quilts over or under the baby or wrapped around the baby can all become hazards, increasing the risk of sleep-related death five-fold [41, 42]. Infants placed in the prone position on soft bedding have a 21-fold increased risk of SIDS [41, 42]. The risk with soft bedding appears to be greatest in infants over 4 months of age [43], so it is especially important to discuss with families as their child gets older and complacency may be setting in regarding objects in the sleep environment.

Although parents are more concerned with their infant getting cold, the greater risk to the baby is over-bundling. Despite making progress in educating families about the dangers of loose and soft bedding, over 55% of families put these materials in the infant's sleep area, and rates are higher in mothers who are young, non-white race/ethnicity or with less than a college education [26, 44]. It is unclear as to whether the risk with head covering is related to hyperthermia, hypoxia, or rebreathing of gases. The studies showing the dangers of head covering generally refer to loose bedding. There are no data regarding hats and increased SIDS risk. However, once infants are able to thermoregulate, there is no need for hats in the sleep environment as they can promote hyperthermia and if dislodged, can theoretically impinge upon the airway.

Well-intentioned parents frequently use quilts and soft bedding to increase their infant's comfort [45]. They also mistakenly use bedding and pillows for infant safety, placing objects around the infant to prevent falling off an adult bed or couch. But as noted above, it is the older infant who is at greatest risk, probably from becoming mobile and getting entangled in the bedding.

Neonatal Abstinence Syndrome (NAS)

Neonatal abstinence syndrome (NAS) refers to a constellation of physiologic and behavioral findings in newborns withdrawing from opioid exposure. Although typically the result of in utero exposure to opioid use (illicit or prescribed), it can occur iatrogenically after a prolonged course of narcotics postnatally. Findings suggestive of NAS include: increased tone, jitteriness, high-pitched cry, excessive fussiness/difficult to console, sweating, fever, mottled skin, excessive sucking, both poor feeding or hyperphagia, vomiting, diarrhea, tachypnea, and seizures. The most common opioids taken by mothers during pregnancy that lead to NAS are buprenorphine +/− naloxone (Subutex/Suboxone) and methadone. The onset of symptoms is related to the half-life of the medication, with symptoms peaking within 3–5 days for buprenorphine and 5–7 days for methadone. Babies exposed to methadone are more likely to require pharmacologic treatment; however, there does not appear to be a relationship between the maternal dose of opioid and the severity of NAS symptoms.

Unfortunately, the incidence of NAS has risen dramatically in the United States with the opioid crisis of the early twenty-first century. Between 2000 and 2009, maternal opioid use increased almost five-fold and in one study, NICU admissions for NAS jumped from 7 to 27 per 1000 live births [46–48].

Parent-Baby Non-separation and Skin-to-Skin Care

One of the keys to successful treatment of NAS is mother-baby non-separation, which is also one of the 10 steps of the Baby Friendly Hospital Initiative and is recommended by the AAP for breastfeeding initiation and success [49, 50]. Studies have demonstrated that increased skin-to-skin care in the maternity setting leads to decreased NAS symptoms and a reduction in pharmacologic intervention with narcotics. As a result, many hospitals are moving away from initial treatment in the NICU setting.

If the infant with NAS can be successfully managed without the need for narcotic medication, the impact is dramatic in terms of both decreased length of hospitalization and cost savings. In addition to mother-baby non-separation and breastfeeding, other non-pharmacologic interventions focus on developmentally sensitive care and promotion of self-regulation, such as: reducing light exposure and excessive noise, avoiding unnecessary handling, swaddling with the arms tucked in, rocking, exposure to white noise and non-nutritive sucking with a pacifier [51–53]. There is some evidence that use of the prone position decreases the severity of neonatal abstinence syndrome scores as well as caloric demands [54].

Management of the infant with NAS is always challenging, and the clinician must be aware of potential conflict between NAS treatment and the need to demonstrate and maintain a safe sleep environment for the infant. Skin-to-skin care is a cornerstone of both normal newborn transition and care of the narcotic-exposed infant. However, as noted in the AAP Clinical Report on Safe Sleep and Skin-to-Skin Care, there are potential harms from infant falls and Sudden Unexpected Postnatal Collapse (SUPC) [55]. Studies have shown infant fall rates in hospitals to range between 1.6 and 4.6 per 10,000 live births [56–58]. Complications from falls can include skull fracture and intracranial hemorrhage. The incidence of SUPC varies widely due to inconsistent definitions between studies but ranges from 2.6 to 133 cases per 100,000 newborns [55]. While SUPC does not always result in infant death, survivors are at high risk for significant neurologic disability at 1 year [59].

Education of staff and new parents on proper technique for skin-to-skin care is paramount to minimizing the risk of injury (see Fig. 10.1). The focus should be on the ABC's of airway, breathing, and circulation. A team in Chicago has coined the phrase "pink and positioned." [60] The airway must be protected so nothing should be obstructing the nose and mouth, and the infant should be positioned such that the face is visible to the parent. The infant should be placed upright between mother's breasts with the head turned to the side, chin horizontal to the body, and the neck flexed slightly less than the sniffing position. The infant should be covered

Position Matters
How to Safely Hold your Baby Skin-to-Skin

For Baby:
Mouth and nose uncovered
Place baby's face above the breasts
Head turned to one side
Neck straight not bent
Make sure the face can be seen
Keep blanket across baby's shoulders, away from the face
Chest to chest with shoulders flat against Mom
Legs flexed

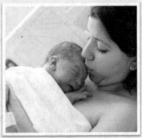

For Parents:
Good support behind Mom's head, back and kness
Mom should be sitting upright not lying back
After breastfeeding, place baby back in upright position

Feeling Sleepy?
Place infant on back in bassinet for Safe Sleep

FIGURE 10.1 Hospital educational poster for proper skin to skin care to prevent hypothermia and sudden unexpected postnatal collapse. (Source: York Hospital, York, PA. Photo source: US Breastfeeding Committee)

but not excessively. If the mother is comfortably clothed, she will keep the baby warm enough. Place a blanket at the baby's shoulders (not above) and tuck the blanket in tightly behind the mother.

Although the baby may be asleep for skin-to-skin care, the mother may NOT. *If the mother is tired, nodding, drowsy or hazy, skin-to-skin should be discontinued or not be initiated.* Staff should be aware of risk factors that have been tied to SUPC, including: first-time mother, lack of knowledge about proper skin-to-skin care, first breastfeeding attempt, mother in episiotomy position, skin-to-skin care without adequate surveillance, overnight hours of 21:00 to 09:00, parents left unattended by the provider after delivery and distractions such as cell phones [55, 59].

In addition to education, healthcare providers should insure adequate, unobtrusive supervision during skin-to-skin care. The Joint Commission has suggested rounding hourly by staff so mothers or other caregivers noted to be drowsy can be assisted to place their newborn in a bassinet [61]. Some have suggested observing every 30 minutes during nighttime and early morning hours for higher-risk dyads [62]. Continuous monitoring is recommended during the first 2 hours after delivery to assure the infant's safe transition to extrauterine life. Up to 37% of SUPC cases occur during this time period. A recent article reported on the use of a bundled intervention including a standardized assessment tool and measurement of oxygen saturation levels with prescribed responses to abnormal values resulting in an elimination of SUPC events from a baseline incidence of 0.54/1000 live births [63].

Rockers, Swings, and Therapeutic Positioning

Although rocking can help with the fussy baby, there may not always be someone available in the hospital or at home to provide this comforting measure. It is common for facilities to use motorized swing devices (such as the mamaRoo®) to provide relief. The challenge with swings is that they must be used only when the infant is awake. These devices are not appropriate for sleeping and have risks similar to those of car seats [64]. Once the baby falls asleep, he must be transferred to a safe sleep surface. And although one can get by with allowing the infant to sleep in the swing while under the continuous monitoring of a NICU setting, it still results in modeling an unsafe sleep environment that might be replicated in the home.

Parents should be made aware of this "therapeutic positioning" early in the hospital course and that as the baby becomes more stable, she will be transitioned to a "safe sleep environment." This is especially true if the need arises for prone positioning. The deeper and longer sleep in the prone position can help with decreased NAS symptoms and calorie consumption. However, as the triple risk model [65] suggests, in the vulnerable infant, the prone position with its deeper sleep may lead to a failure of arousal from an environmental threat, resulting in an increased risk of sudden and unexpected death.

Finally, infant safe sleep education must be a priority with families caring for the infant with NAS. Many of these families will be involved with Child Protective Services. One study found that the rate of SIDS was more than 3 times as great among infants reported for possible maltreatment [66]. Also, many of these mothers remain on maintenance therapy for their substance use disorder. These medications result in drowsiness that greatly increases the risk of SIDS while bedsharing [67].

Upper Respiratory Tract Infections and Fever

Due to their immature immune systems, it is very common for infants to acquire minor colds, gastrointestinal infections, and other febrile illnesses. The average child has between 6 and 8 colds during the first year of life, and 10–15% will have at least 12 infections per year. Any illness can create stress and worry for new parents. Parents want to keep their children safe, prevent suffering, and provide comfort. Unfortunately, misguided efforts to protect and console children can actually increase the risk of harm. Providing comfort for a sick child is frequently given as a reason by parents for bedsharing, with the belief that their own vigilance is the only way that they can keep their infant safe and that the close proximity of bedsharing allows them to maintain vigilance, even while sleeping [68–70]. The potential dangers of bedsharing have been discussed elsewhere in this book (Chap. 6); however, there are particular concerns with the febrile child. The amount of clothing or blankets covering an infant (which are often increased in a bedsharing scenario) and the room temperature are associated with an increased risk of SIDS [71–73]. It is unclear if overheating is an independent risk factor or an association with the increased risk of SIDS and suffocation from potentially asphyxiating objects in the sleep environment such as loose blankets.

Some parents also want to elevate the infant's head by using an inclined sleep surface or something similar because they perceive that it will be easier for the infant to breathe. As mentioned in Chap. 8, it takes more muscle strength for an infant to lie on an incline and, because of the larger head:body ratio, it is more difficult to maintain a clear airway on an inclined sleep surface [74]. Babies may fatigue more easily. Thus, a flat surface remains the safest for an infant with an upper respiratory infection.

Infection, even without fever, has been noted to be commonly associated with SIDS in case-control studies. A causal role has been suggested, because in approximately half of SIDS cases the infant had a recent minor infection [75]. Autopsy frequently reveals mild tracheobronchial inflammation, altered cytokine levels and serum immunoglobulins and microbial isolates [76, 77]. Although some cases of SIDS may be directly caused by infection, it is possible that a minor infection may represent an extrinsic risk factor in the triple risk hypothesis that affects the vulnerable infant at a critical time in development.

Regardless of the multiple mechanisms by which infection may make the infant more vulnerable to SIDS, clinicians should take the opportunity to reinforce safe sleep messaging during a time of illness. It is important to balance such messaging to not panic parents who are already concerned with their child's illness. The focus in this situation is on preventing additional risk from further temperature elevation as well as the many potential risks from bedsharing.

Conditions with Potential Airway Compromise

Although uncommon, there are congenital and acquired conditions that may leave an infant vulnerable to airway compromise. This, in turn, may increase the infant's risk of SIDS/asphyxia either directly through airway obstruction or impaired ventilation or indirectly through non-supine positioning or the need for positioners or soft bedding. The former would include conditions such as tracheobronchomalacia and subglottic stenosis, while the latter would include congenital myotonic dystrophy and hypoxic-ischemic encephalopathy.

As an example, care for the infant with Pierre Robin sequence can be particularly challenging. In the sequence the midline cleft palate allows the tongue to lay more posterior and limits the proper growth of the mandible, resulting in retrognathia. When the baby lays supine, the tongue can fall further back into the pharynx leading to airway obstruction. In the 40% of cases that are severe, infants will require an inpatient surgical intervention, either mandibular distraction osteogenesis, tongue-lip adhesion or tracheostomy, resulting in a stable airway in supine position at discharge [78]. For infants with mild disease who do not have significant airway obstruction and can maintain normal ventilation and oxygenation in the supine sleep position, families can be instructed to follow standard safe sleep recommendations.

The challenge for the clinician is the infant who is not severe enough for surgical intervention but is not stable in the supine position. In this scenario, it may be necessary to instruct the family to maintain the baby in the lateral or prone position for sleep. This could be considered analogous to the rare situation where the risk of death from GERD outweighs the risk of SIDS, such as with a grade IV laryngeal cleft [21]. Although monitors are not recommended to reduce the risk of SIDS, home monitoring devices, including pulse-oximeters may be appropriate for children at risk of central or obstructive apnea or hypoventilation, to alert caregivers to the possibility of potentially dangerous respiratory compromise when not under direct observation. These decisions should be individualized based on the clinical situation and the psychosocial dynamics of the family.

Vignette Follow-Up

Let's return to our clinical scenario. There are numerous theories for successful healthcare behavior change. Common themes amongst the theories include having empathetic, nonjudgmental conversations, allowing parents to drive the conversation by asking most of the questions and guiding them toward coming up with their own solutions that will work in their day to day life. It's important to ask permission to have the conversation about infant sleep safety.

Now that we have listened to Linda's story, we can start with empathetic observation, validation and positive reinforcement for both mother and her support person: "Linda, thank you so much for sharing your story with me. I can see that this has not been an easy journey for you and Starr, but she looks very healthy on her exam today and you are doing a wonderful job taking care of her. It's great to see your mom here with you. Having family and friends available can be so helpful in dealing with the stress and lack of sleep that comes with a new baby in the home."

"You've brought up some important concerns regarding Starr's fussiness and feedings. If it's okay with you, I would like to review some information about reflux and feeding practices, calming fussy babies and maintaining a safe sleep environment." After Linda gives us permission, we can review what is being done for Starr's reflux to make sure the family is taking advantage of all available treatment modalities. This would also be a good time to review the benefits of breastfeeding and congratulate Linda on her efforts. Reviewing the baby's growth curve with the family can provide reassurance that the feedings are going well.

It is also important to gently educate the grandmother since she is an important support to Linda and may be a central node of influence on Linda and her decisions on how Starr is cared for. We can introduce the idea of putting an endpoint on Starr's course of Omeprazole and make note of the fact that longer courses of the medication have been associated with increased risk of infection and increased risk of bone fractures when children get more mobile.

We will want to provide anticipatory guidance in reviewing what techniques the family is using to help control Starr's fussiness. It is important to acknowledge that although Starr is over the worst of her withdrawal, it is common for babies with NAS to have some persistent symptoms for weeks to months after discharge from the hospital. For the skeptical family, it may be beneficial to have them view some on-line examples of parents using the calming techniques of swaddling, white noise/shushing, swinging, etc. Since any technique may not be successful every time, there should be discussion of developing a safety plan for respite and avoiding abusive head trauma, formerly known as Shaken Baby Syndrome.

No newborn visit should be considered complete without a review of infant sleep safety. This author likes to initiate the discussion with the open-ended question of what sleep arrangements have been made for the baby. This will allow for more dialogue rather than yes/no responses. Praise and positive reinforcement should be given for behaviors that are consistent with the safe sleep recommendations. For behaviors that place the infant at risk, the clinician should explore the reasoning behind the behavior in a non-judgmental way, such as asking, "Help me understand why you place your baby on the tummy to sleep." Appropriate education can be brought into the discussion.

In our vignette, the discussion about reflux can provide a natural transition into safe sleep since even infants with reflux should be placed on the back to sleep. The anatomic drawings can be incorporated into the education as well as a discussion of the success of the back to sleep campaign in reducing SIDS deaths by over 50%. Mothers are very focused on social norms and may be positively influenced by knowing that over 75% of mothers routinely place their infants on the back for sleep [24–26].

Finally, it is important to remember that family members are part of the mother's social network and may be very influential regarding infant care issues. Making sure these influencers are on the same page regarding infant sleep safety can significantly reduce barriers to appropriate behaviors. When family members (especially the grandmother) are present, their importance as a resource and helper should be recognized. Again, the discussion should be non-judgmental. It is important to acknowledge the ways of the past and that older ways of doing things were appropriate at the time. This author likes to make comparisons with obsolete technologies, such as traditional phones and VCRs. We have adapted to newer and better technology. Medicine is no different- we want to use the latest technology and research to drive best practices, including best infant sleep practices to keep babies healthy and out of harm's way.

Clinical Pearls

GER(D):

- GER is normal and should be differentiated from GERD.
- GER is self-limited and requires more parental reassurance than intervention.
- GERD should NOT be treated with inclined positioning of the infant.
- GERD should be treated in a step-wise fashion.

- Infants should sleep supine regardless of GER(D), except for the rare instance that the risk of death from reflux is greater than the risk of death from SUID.
- The use of visual education tools (cross-sectional anatomic images of the infant in supine and prone position) can significantly enhance family understanding of the benefits of supine positioning in the face of GER(D).

NG Tubes:

- There is no evidence that infants receiving NG or orogastric feedings are at increased risk of aspiration if placed in the supine position.

Hypothermia:

- Hypothermia in the preterm infant is associated with increased morbidity and mortality.
- Heat loss can occur through radiant, conductive, convective, and evaporative mechanisms.
- Skin-to-skin care should be initiated immediately after birth in healthy newborns.
- Over-bundling is associated with an increased risk of SIDS.
- Room temperature should be comfortable for a lightly clothed adult. Infants should have one additional layer of clothing.
- Infant clothing/sleepwear or wearable blankets are preferable to loose blankets or quilts which can lead to head covering and suffocation risk.

NAS:

- After hospital discharge, infants exposed to narcotics in utero are frequently fussy, placing them at risk for exposure to unsafe sleep environments to promote calming and sleep (prone position, bedsharing).
- Extra anticipatory guidance should be provided regarding techniques for calming fussy babies, including: skin-to-skin care, infant massage, the 5 S's (swaddling, swinging, shushing, sucking, and side carry).

- The use of swings can be effective in calming fussy babies, however parents must be vigilant in transitioning their infant to a safe sleep environment once they fall asleep.
- Parents on medications that impair alertness should be reminded of the extreme danger of sharing a sleep surface (bedsharing) with their baby.
- Help parents of NAS infants create a back-up plan for child care help if the infant becomes especially fussy. Respite is critical to avoiding situations that could lead to an unsafe sleep environment or abusive head trauma.

Viral Respiratory Illnesses/Fever:

- Viral illnesses and fever are very common during the first year of life.
- Bedsharing and use of inclined sleep surfaces are not recommended at any time, and particularly when the infant is ill.
- Overheating and/or head covering have been associated with an increased risk of SIDS.
- It is important at sick visits to review infant sleep safety, especially warning parents of the dangers of bedsharing, overheating, and head covering.

Conditions with Potential Airway Compromise:

- Although uncommon, there are infants that require the use of non-supine sleep positioning due to abnormal anatomy or physiology impacting respiration.
- Monitors are not recommended to reduce the risk of SIDS; however, monitoring devices, including pulse-oximeters can be used in children at risk for central or obstructive apnea, to alert caregivers to the possibility of potentially dangerous respiratory compromise when not under direct observation.

References

1. Nelson SP, Chen EH, Syniar GM, Christoffel KK. Prevalence of symptoms of gastroesophageal reflux during infancy. A pediatric practice-based survey. Pediatric Practice Research Group. Arch Pediatr Adolesc Med. 1997;151(6):569–72.

2. Eichenwald EC, Committee On F, Newborn. Diagnosis and management of gastroesophageal reflux in preterm infants. Pediatrics. 2018;142(1):e20181061.

3. Kuribayashi S, Massey BT, Hafeezullah M, Perera L, Hussaini SQ, Tatro L, et al. Terminating motor events for TLESR are influenced by the presence and distribution of refluxate. Am J Physiol Gastrointest Liver Physiol. 2009;297(1):G71–5.

4. Torrico S, Kern M, Aslam M, Narayanan S, Kannappan A, Ren J, et al. Upper esophageal sphincter function during gastroesophageal reflux events revisited. Am J Physiol Gastrointest Liver Physiol. 2000;279(2):G262–7.

5. Kim HI, Hong SJ, Han JP, Seo JY, Hwang KH, Maeng HJ, et al. Specific movement of esophagus during transient lower esophageal sphincter relaxation in gastroesophageal reflux disease. J Neurogastroenterol Motil. 2013;19(3):332–7.

6. Neu J, Douglas-Escobar M, Fucile S. Gastrointestinal development: implications for infant feeding. In: Duggan CP, Watkins JB, Koletzko B, Walker WA, Mehta L, editors. Nutrition in pediatrics. 5th ed. Shelton: People's Medical Publishing House; 2016. p. 387–98.

7. Lightdale JR, Gremse DA. Gastroesophageal reflux: management guidance for the pediatrician. Pediatrics. 2013;131(5): e1684–95.

8. Bhat RY, Rafferty GF, Hannam S, Greenough A. Acid gastroesophageal reflux in convalescent preterm infants: effect of posture and relationship to apnea. Pediatr Res. 2007;62(5):620–3.

9. Corvaglia L, Rotatori R, Ferlini M, Aceti A, Ancora G, Faldella G. The effect of body positioning on gastroesophageal reflux in premature infants: evaluation by combined impedance and pH monitoring. J Pediatr. 2007;151(6):591–6, 6.e1.

10. Omari TI, Rommel N, Staunton E, Lontis R, Goodchild L, Haslam RR, et al. Paradoxical impact of body positioning on gastroesophageal reflux and gastric emptying in the premature neonate. J Pediatr. 2004;145(2):194–200.

11. van Wijk MP, Benninga MA, Dent J, Lontis R, Goodchild L, McCall LM, et al. Effect of body position changes on postprandial gastroesophageal reflux and gastric emptying in the healthy premature neonate. J Pediatr. 2007;151(6):585–90, 90.e1–2.

12. Orenstein SR, Whitington PF, Orenstein DM. The infant seat as treatment for gastroesophageal reflux. N Engl J Med. 1983;309(13):760–3.

13. Shuren J. In: Administration USFaD, editor. Letter to manufacturers concerning medical claims about infant sleep positioners: devices can create risk of suffocation. Washington, DC: US Food and Drug Administration; 2010.

14. Peachman RR. Fisher-Price rock 'n play sleeper should be recalled, consumer reports says. Consumer Rep. 2019.

15. U.S. Consumer product safety commission, safety standard for infant sleep products. Fed Register 2019;84(218):60649–60963.

16. Rahal PS, Wright RA. Transdermal nicotine and gastroesophageal reflux. Am J Gastroenterol. 1995;90(6):919–21.

17. Pandolfino JE, Kahrilas PJ. Smoking and gastro-oesophageal reflux disease. Eur J Gastroenterol Hepatol. 2000;12(8):837–42.

18. Djeddi D, Stephan-Blanchard E, Leke A, Ammari M, Delanaud S, Lemaire-Hurtel AS, et al. Effects of smoking exposure in infants on gastroesophageal reflux as a function of the sleep-wakefulness state. J Pediatr. 2018;201:147–53.

19. Salvatore S, Vandenplas Y. Gastroesophageal reflux and cow milk allergy: is there a link? Pediatrics. 2002;110(5):972–84.

20. Malloy MH. Trends in postneonatal aspiration deaths and reclassification of sudden infant death syndrome: impact of the "Back to sleep" program. Pediatrics. 2002;109(4):661–5.

21. Moon RY. Task Force on Sudden Infant Death Syndrome, SIDS and other sleep-related infant deaths: evidence base for 2016 updated recommendations for a safe infant sleeping environment. Pediatrics. 2016;138(5):e20162940.

22. Byard RW, Beal S. Gastric aspiration and sleeping position in infancy and early childhood. J Paediatr Child Health. 2000;36:403–5.

23. Tablizo MA, Jacinto P, Parsley D, Chen ML, Ramanathan R, Keens TG. Supine sleeping position does not cause clinical aspiration in neonates in hospital newborn nurseries. Arch Pediatr Adolesc Med. 2007;161(5):507–10.

24. Moon RY, Carlin RF, Cornwell B, Mathews A, Oden RP, Cheng YI, et al. Implications of Mothers' social networks for risky infant sleep practices. J Pediatr. 2019;212:151–8.e2.
25. Colson E, Geller NL, Heeren T, Corwin MJ. Factors associated with choice of infant sleep position. Pediatrics. 2017;140(3):e20170596.
26. Hirai AH, Kortsmit K, Kaplan L, Reiney E, Warner L, Parks SE, et al. Prevalence and factors associated with safe infant sleep practices. Pediatrics. 2019;144(5). e20191286
27. Peter CS, Wiechers C, Bohnhorst B, Silny J, Poets CF. Influence of nasogastric tubes on gastroesophageal reflux in preterm infants: a multiple intraluminal impedance study. J Pediatr. 2002;141(2):277–9.
28. Mendes TB, Mezzacappa MA, Toro AA, Ribeiro JD. Risk factors for gastroesophageal reflux disease in very low birth weight infants with bronchopulmonary dysplasia. J Pediatr. 2008;84(2):154–9.
29. Murthy SV, Funderburk A, Abraham S, Epstein M, DiPalma J, Aghai ZH. Nasogastric feeding tubes may not contribute to gastroesophageal reflux in preterm infants. Am J Perinatol. 2018;35(7):643–7.
30. Stavis R. Hypothermia in neonates 2019. Updated July 2019. Available from: https://www.merckmanuals.com/professional/pediatrics/perinatal-problems/hypothermia-in-neonates.
31. Wilson E, Maier RF, Norman M, Misselwitz B, Howell EA, Zeitlin J, et al. Admission hypothermia in very preterm infants and neonatal mortality and morbidity. J Pediatr. 2016;175:61–7. e4
32. Laptook AR, Bell EF, Shankaran S, Boghossian NS, Wyckoff MH, Kandefer S, et al. Admission temperature and associated mortality and morbidity among moderately and extremely preterm infants. J Pediatr. 2018;192:53–9.e2.
33. Kilpatrick SJ, Papile L-A, editors. American Academy of pediatric committee on fetus and newborn and American College of Obstetricians and Gynecologists, guidelines for perinatal care. 8th ed. Elk Grove Village: American Academy of Pediatrics; 2017.
34. World Health Organization, Maternal and Newborn Health/Safe Motherhood. Thermal protection of the newborn: a practical guide. 2016.
35. Nimbalkar SM, Patel VK, Patel DV, Nimbalkar AS, Sethi A, Phatak A. Effect of early skin-to-skin contact following normal

delivery on incidence of hypothermia in neonates more than 1800 g: randomized control trial. J Perinatol. 2014;34(5):364–8.

36. Moore ER, Anderson GC. Randomized controlled trial of very early mother-infant skin-to-skin contact and breastfeeding status. J Midwifery Womens Health. 2007;52(2):116–25.

37. Colson ER, Bergman DM, Shapiro E, Leventhal JH. Position for newborn sleep: associations with parents' perceptions of their nursery experience. Birth. 2001;28(4):249–53.

38. Goodstein MH, Bell T, Krugman SD. Improving infant sleep safety through a comprehensive hospital-based program. Clin Pediatr (Phila). 2015;54(3):212–21.

39. Mason B, Ahlers-Schmidt CR, Schunn C. Improving safe sleep environments for well newborns in the hospital setting. Clin Pediatr (Phila). 2013;52(10):969–75.

40. Kellams A, Parker MG, Geller NL, Moon RY, Colson ER, Drake E, et al. Todays baby quality improvement: safe sleep teaching and role modeling in 8 US Maternity Units. Pediatrics. 2017;140(5). e20171816

41. Hauck FR, Herman SM, Donovan M, Iyasu S, Merrick Moore C, Donoghue E, et al. Sleep environment and the risk of sudden infant death syndrome in an urban population: the Chicago Infant Mortality Study. Pediatrics. 2003;111(5 Part 2):1207–14.

42. Scheers NJ, Dayton CM, Kemp JS. Sudden infant death with external airways covered: case-comparison study of 206 deaths in the United States. Arch Pediatr Adolesc Med. 1998;152:540–7.

43. Colvin JD, Collie-Akers V, Schunn C, Moon RY. Sleep environment risks for younger and older infants. Pediatrics. 2014;134(2):e406–12.

44. Shapiro-Mendoza CK, Colson ER, Willinger M, Rybin DV, Camperlengo L, Corwin MJ. Trends in infant bedding use: national infant sleep position study, 1993–2010. Pediatrics. 2015;135(1):10–7.

45. Ajao TI, Oden RP, Joyner BL, Moon RY. Decisions of black parents about infant bedding and sleep surfaces: a qualitative study. Pediatrics. 2011;128(3):494–502.

46. Patrick SW, Schumacher RE, Benneyworth BD, Krans EE, McAllister JM, Davis MM. Neonatal abstinence syndrome and associated health care expenditures: United States, 2000–2009. JAMA. 2012;307(18):1934–40.

47. Patrick SW, Davis MM, Lehmann CU, Cooper WO. Increasing incidence and geographic distribution of neonatal abstinence syndrome: United States 2009 to 2012. J Perinatol. 2015;35(8):650–5.

48. Ko JY, Patrick SW, Tong VT, Patel R, Lind JN, Barfield WD. Incidence of neonatal abstinence syndrome – 28 states, 1999–2013. MMWR Morb Mortal Wkly Rep. 2016;65(31):799–802.

49. McKnight S, Coo H, Davies G, Holmes B, Newman A, Newton L, et al. Rooming-in for infants at risk of neonatal abstinence syndrome. Am J Perinatol. 2016;33(5):495–501.

50. Holmes AV, Atwood EC, Whalen B, Beliveau J, Jarvis JD, Matulis JC, et al. Rooming-in to treat neonatal abstinence syndrome: improved family-centered care at lower cost. Pediatrics. 2016;137(6). e20152929

51. Maguire D. Care of the infant with neonatal abstinence syndrome: strength of the evidence. J Perinat Neonatal Nurs. 2014;28(3):204–11; quiz E3–4.

52. Wachman EM, Schiff DM, Silverstein M. Neonatal abstinence syndrome: advances in diagnosis and treatment. JAMA. 2018;319(13):1362–74.

53. Grossman M, Seashore C, Holmes AV. Neonatal abstinence syndrome management: a review of recent evidence. Rev Recent Clin Trials. 2017;12(4):226–32.

54. Maichuk GT, Zahorodny W, Marshall R. Use of positioning to reduce the severity of neonatal narcotic withdrawal syndrome. J Perinatol. 1999;19(7):510–3.

55. Feldman-Winter L, Goldsmith JP, Committee On Fetus and Newborn, Task Force On Sudden Infant Death Syndrome. Safe sleep and skin-to-skin care in the neonatal period for healthy term newborns. Pediatrics. 2016;138(3). e20161889

56. Helsley L, McDonald JV, Stewart VT. Addressing in-hospital "falls" of newborn infants. Jt Comm J Qual Patient Saf. 2010;36(7):327–33.

57. Loyal J, Pettker CM, Raab CA, O'Mara E, Lipkind HS. Newborn falls in a large tertiary academic center over 13 years. Hosp Pediatr. 2018; e20180021

58. Monson SA, Henry E, Lambert DK, Schmutz N, Christensen RD. In-hospital falls of newborn infants: data from a multihospital health care system. Pediatrics. 2008;122(2):e277–80.

59. Herlenius E, Kuhn P. Sudden unexpected postnatal collapse of newborn infants: a review of cases, definitions, risks, and preventive measures. Transl Stroke Res. 2013;4(2):236–47.

60. Garofalo NA, Pellerite MR, Goodstein MH, Paul DA, Hageman JR. Sudden Unexpected Postnatal Collapse (SUPC): one newborn death is too many: current concepts. Neonatol Today. 2019(February):55–7.

61. The Joint Commission, Division of Healthcare Improvement. Quick Safety. Preventing newborn falls and drops. 2018.
62. Gaffey AD. Fall prevention in our healthiest patients: assessing risk and preventing injury for moms and babies. J Healthc Risk Manag. 2015;34(3):37–40.
63. Paul DA, Johnson D, Goldstein ND, Pearlman SA. Development of a single-center quality bundle to prevent sudden unexpected postnatal collapse. J Perinatol. 2019;39(7):1008–13.
64. Batra EK, Midgett JD, Moon RY. Hazards associated with sitting and carrying devices for children two years and younger. J Pediatr. 2015;167(1):183–7.
65. Filiano JJ, Kinney HC. A perspective on neuropathologic findings in victims of the sudden infant death syndrome: the triple-risk model. Biol Neonate. 1994;65:194–7.
66. Putnam-Hornstein E, Schneiderman JU, Cleves MA, Magruder J, Krous HF. A prospective study of sudden unexpected infant death after reported maltreatment. J Pediatr. 2014;164(1): 142–8.
67. Carpenter R, McGarvey C, Mitchell EA, Tappin DM, Vennemann MM, Smuk M, et al. Bed sharing when parents do not smoke: is there a risk of SIDS? An individual level analysis of five major case-control studies. BMJ Open. 2013;3(5):e002299.
68. Hauck FR, Signore C, Fein SB, Raju TN. Infant sleeping arrangements and practices during the first year of life. Pediatrics. 2008;122(Suppl 2):S113–20.
69. Ward TC. Reasons for mother-infant bed-sharing: a systematic narrative synthesis of the literature and implications for future research. Matern Child Health J. 2015;19(3):675–90.
70. Joyner BL, Oden R, Ajao TI, Moon R. Where should my baby sleep? A qualitative study of African-American infant sleep location decisions. J Natl Med Assoc. 2010;102(10):881–9.
71. Fleming P, Gilbert R, Azaz Y, Berry PJ, Rudd PT, Stewart A, et al. Interaction between bedding and sleeping position in the sudden infant death syndrome: a population based case-control study. BMJ. 1990;301:85–9.
72. Ponsonby A-L, Dwyer T, Gibbons LE, Cochrane JA, Jones ME, McCall MJ. Thermal environment and sudden infant death syndrome: case-control study. BMJ. 1992;304:277–82.
73. Ponsonby A-L, Dwyer T, Gibbons LE, Cochrane JA, Wang Y-G. Factors potentiating the risk of sudden infant death syndrome associated with the prone position. N Engl J Med. 1993;329:377–82.

74. Mannen EM, Carroll J, Bumpass DB, Rabenhorst B, Whitaker B, Wang J, et al. Biomechanical analysis of inclined sleep products. Little Rock: University of Arkansas; 2019.
75. Kinney HC, Thach BT. The sudden infant death syndrome. N Engl J Med. 2009;361(8):795–805.
76. Vege A, Ole Rognum T. Sudden infant death syndrome, infection and inflammatory responses. FEMS Immunol Med Microbiol. 2004;42(1):3–10.
77. Weber MA, Klein NJ, Hartley JC, Lock PE, Malone M, Sebire NJ. Infection and sudden unexpected death in infancy: a systematic retrospective case review. Lancet. 2008;371(9627):1848–53.
78. Insalaco LF, Scott AR. Peripartum management of neonatal Pierre Robin sequence. Clin Perinatol. 2018;45(4):717–35.

Chapter 11
If the Unthinkable Happens: Families After SUID

Richard D. Goldstein

Clinical Vignette

Bill and Ayanna woke in surprise that their four-month-old son hadn't cried yet for his morning breastfeeding. Then they discovered Zach dead in his crib. "This makes no sense. There was nothing wrong with him!" they recounted later. They had placed him in the supine position with a loose blanket in a portable crib beside their bed, after his 3 AM breastfeeding. He was discovered prone, head to his side, with his blanket beneath him. After attempts at CPR, emergency response, and transfer to the local hospital, Zach was declared dead in their local emergency room.

In the ER, the staff was sympathetic. The parents were given time to hold Zach but their last moments with him occurred under observation. Bill and Ayanna were separated for interviews with social workers and child protective services. Questions were asked about what happened. They were asked about their 4-year-old daughter and were told that social services needed assurances about her safety. They were

R. D. Goldstein (✉)
Robert's Program on Sudden Unexpected Death in Pediatrics,
Division of General Pediatrics, Department of Pediatrics,
Boston Children's Hospital and Harvard Medical School,
Boston, MA, USA
e-mail: Richard.goldstein@childrens.harvard.edu

© Springer Nature Switzerland AG 2020
R. Y. Moon (ed.), *Infant Safe Sleep*,
https://doi.org/10.1007/978-3-030-47542-0_11

warned that her removal from their home was a possibility and a social worker from child protective services was sent to interview her. When they returned home for their first private moment to console one another, Bill and Ayanna returned to death scene investigators.

Their pediatrician attended the funeral and her office sent a sincere sympathy card, but she felt ill prepared to advise the family about what happened or what to expect in the investigation. After months with little contact from the medical examiners, a death certificate arrived by mail. The cause and manner of death were listed as "undetermined". Ayanna was unable to read it or to talk about it. Bill found the document unreadable because of its language and what it described. During this time, the couple was overwhelmed by grief, self-questioning and isolation. Zach's nursery and his things remain virtually untouched.

The preceding chapters presented information about recognizing and navigating sleep position and environmental risks. Unfortunately, infants continue to die from unexplained, sleep-related causes with disturbing frequency. Whether an infant died with or without risk factors, the family's health care providers will find themselves as the clinicians to a terribly bereft family at a time when those risk factors matter in a very different way. The focus of this chapter is on the family experiences, likely responses, available resources, and the clinician's role following an infant's death. The intent is to increase the reader's understanding of this experience from a parent's perspective and offer practical ways to offer help.

Family Experience

As the above scenario illustrates, a sudden and unexpected infant death involves family tragedy, child protection concerns, and a mandated investigation. At a moment of inestimable, disorienting loss, young parents generally find themselves dealing with their first death, their first interactions with forensic and public safety systems, and the startling lack of options for explanation and support. The first pause after discovering their deceased infant generally becomes the beginning of witness interviews and the initiation of an emotionally trying process that may seem to prioritize the establishment of wrongdoing. Available supports and services to help distressed parents and families following the unanticipated and profound loss of their baby are less obvious.

Gathering information about the deceased infant begins when resuscitative efforts are discontinued and the infant's death is declared. From the investigative and child safety perspective, this is understandable. Recall bias is a concern in the confusion and high emotions after the death. From the perspective of an acutely bereaved parent, it can feel intrusive, unkind and overwhelming, even when they recognize the reasons for this approach. Research on parent outcomes of grief severity and regret, as well as parent preferences, shows the importance of affording the time and the respect for acutely bereaved parents to hold their child and say goodbye [1].

Practices vary by jurisdiction, but great strides have been made to provide uniform data gathering and training for those responsible to collect it [2]. This occurs in different phases, with first responders and law enforcement typically at the first point of contact, and medical (sometimes), child protective, and forensic professionals later. This data gathering works best when the response is coordinated and carried out in a way that balances supportive interactions for the family with the needs of the investigation [3].

In almost any setting, authorities and statutes mandate an investigation into the cause and manner of an infant's death when it is unexpected. That investigation begins immediately with a focused physical examination. This examination is crucial to document postmortem changes, although the infant is rarely seen as they were first discovered. The initial physical examination also looks for any physical evidence of child abuse or criminal neglect that may have been contributory. "Witness interviews" occur promptly, with recognition that the recall of a shocked and acutely bereaved parent or care-giver may lack the precision investigators might prefer. It is recommended practice to interview parents separately, and special attention is paid to eliciting separate uninfluenced recollections from the "placers" and the "finders" of the infant for the last sleep period, if they are different people. During the witness interviews, the topics critical for the investigation include details of the last time the infant was seen alive and of the infant's discovery, the infant's 72 hours preceding the death, family demographics, past medical history including recent illnesses, diet and vaccinations, and a pregnancy history [4]. The occurrence of any sudden or unexpected infant or childhood death in first- to third-degree relatives is also informative. Generally, the deceased infant is then transferred to the medical examiner or coroner's office for a complete autopsy. Parents usually have questions they feel reluctant to ask about what happens to their babies when they are taken to the morgue.

Medical examiners and coroners are entrusted with determining why the infant died. There is a general consensus about what constitutes a complete investigation following sudden unexpected infant deaths [5]. It is generally comprised of a thorough historical review of medical and social service (when present) records, a review of the details of the death scene and witness reports, a general external and internal autopsy examination, blood cultures and viral swabs, toxicology, and histology. The death scene review is conducted by a death investigator or their representative at the place where the infant was found. It is advocated that this review includes a doll re-enactment of the events and questions about the general health, recent health, and routines of the infant. Within the forensic community, there is a consensus about the value of doll re-enactments. Although they are usually performed with sensitivity, many parents report that these graphic re-enactments are quite triggering of emotional distress.

A general autopsy is usually performed within 72 hours of the death, often within 24 hours. The autopsy involves a detailed external and internal examination, along with radiology, toxicology, and histology, in all cases. Most assessments also include microbiology testing and clinical chemistry testing. Neuropathology can be revealing and involves brain fixation with formalin, which can take 2–4 weeks before the brain is ready for sectioning. Genetic studies are increasingly pursued as part of the initial autopsy, subject to the resources and protocols of each medical examiner's office. At a minimum, samples for genetics are gathered at the autopsy, allowing elective testing according to autopsy findings or parental preferences. When family history suggests a potential genetic etiology, e.g., a family history of life-limiting or life-shortening cardiac arrhythmias, "panels" of genes identified in reference to specific etiologies may be obtained, with results potentially available in a matter of days. A more openly diagnostic approach involving whole exome sequencing may also be pursued. The sequencing generally takes 8–10 weeks and can be followed with an automated report. More exploratory, research-related genetic curation will take longer. Rapid exomes are available as quickly as within 50 hours [6], although such technology is generally beyond the resources of most medical examiner systems. State laws may prohibit such testing without parental permission or may not fund genetic testing.

Parents may be comforted to know that their infant is treated with tenderness and respect during the autopsy, and that medical examiners are often extremely moved by the unfortunate fate of the infant. Religious and burial practices are invariably accommodated; it is extremely helpful for parents to make medical examiners aware of cultural or religious death practices. The established standard set by the National Association of Medical Examiners for the time necessary for the completion of a death certificate and autopsy is within 90 days [7]. Medical examiners often make themselves available to bereaved families for any questions, and this can include an in-person conference with the families. In many jurisdictions, the family must initiate this contact.

- Send a letter of condolence to the parents.
- Make a bereavement call to check in with the family.
- Offer to sit down with the family to talk about what is known about sudden and unexpected infant death, and about the predicament they find themselves in.
- Stay involved and offer to help the family investigate cause.
- Make a note of the child's death in the chart for when they come in for another child's visit.
- Use the child's name.

FIGURE 11.1 Suggestions for helping a newly bereaved family

The infant's primary care providers may first learn about the infant's death when they receive an inquiry about child protective concerns. Sometimes they are notified when the infant is in the emergency room or in the home. Going to the location to support the family during this very difficult time is a great service (Fig. 11.1).

Primary care providers usually respond with sympathy at the news of the infant's death, but it is important to frankly recognize how little is typically offered. This may be due to the rarity of the outcome, the feeling that the medical aspects of the case are issues involving the medicolegal system and outside of their area of expertise, or the lack of training or education about what a potential role might be. Even when a provider is motivated to assist the family, there is no broadly disseminated clinical model centered on families and their experiences after a sudden and unexpected infant death [8]. In many cases, this means that many of the parents' questions or concerns are never heard. Parents may resort to conducting online searches to answer questions like what lividity is, what the frothy blood-tinged secretions they observed on their infant's face were, or whether SIDS is suffocation, often with disturbing results (See Fig. 11.2a, b).

Additionally, mothers who have been breastfeeding may find it helpful to consult a lactation consultant for assistance with the management of breast engorgement and milk suppression.

a can I get arrested for SIDS?   🎤 🔍

🔍 All   📰 News   🛒 Shopping   🖼 Images   ▶ Videos   ⋮ More   Settings   Tools

About 211,000 results (0.63 seconds)

Sudden Infant Death Syndrome Laws - Ncsl
https://www.ncsl.org › research › health › sudden-infant-death-syndrome-l... ▾
The team is **charged** with the development, maintenance, and provision of ... If the coroner finds
the cause of death to be **SIDS**, he **shall** notify the director of the ...

People also ask	
Can you get arrested for SIDS?	∨
Do police investigate SIDS?	∨
Can you stop SIDS while it's happening?	∨
What happens when a baby dies suddenly?	∨

Feedback

Sudden Infant Death Syndrome and the Charges Parents May ...
https://www.grgblaw.com › wisconsin-trial-lawyers › sudden-infant-death-... ▾
Jan 5, 2016 - Many **SIDS** deaths remain a mystery. Unfortunately, some **SIDS** deaths end up
resulting in criminal charges for parents or caretakers, compounding tragedy on top of tragedy. ...
Other cases involve parents/caregivers who seem to **have** done everything possible to reduce
the risk to their babies.

Yes, It Is Possible to Be Charged with Manslaughter If Your ...
https://www.everydayfamily.com › blog › yes-you-can-be-charged-with-m... ▾
SIDS is an absolute terror for parents everywhere, and it **can** also **be** a double-edged sword.

Parents: 'Our baby died - then the police arrived' | Life and ...
https://www.theguardian.com › may › familyandrelationships.children ▾
May 25, 2005 - ... died in her sleep, the last thing her parents expected was to **be** arrested. ...
baby **could** just die so I was convinced that I must **be** responsible in some way. ... **Sudden infant
death syndrome (Sids)**, or cot death, is the most ...

SIDS: Many Deaths No Longer A Mystery : NPR
https://www.npr.org › 2011/07/15 › rethinking-sids-many-deaths-no-longer-...
Jul 15, 2011 - Many cases once thought to **be sudden infant death syndrome** are now ... The
baby **could be** too hot if you notice sweating, damp hair, flushed ...

Mother's prosecution in accidental suffocation death of ...

FIGURE 11.2 Results from Google searches that are frequently conducted by parents who have lost a baby suddenly and unexpectedly

b   do parents kill their babies in SIDS?   🎤 🔍

Q All   🖻 News   🖾 Images   ▶ Videos   ⬮ Shopping   ⋮ More   Settings   Tools
___

About 478,000 results (0.54 seconds)

Ten Percent of SIDS Cases are Murder — or are They? - NCBI
https://www.ncbi.nlm.nih.gov › pmc › articles › PMC6474533 ▾
by CM Milroy - 2017 - Cited by 3 - Related articles
Jun 1, 2017 - The term sudden infant death syndrome (SIDS) was introduced in ... He stated that
more mothers had confessed to killing their child than he ...
Abstract · Introduction · Discussion · Conclusion

Murder misdiagnosed as SIDS - Archives of Disease in - The ...
https://adc.bmj.com › content
by J Stanton - 2001 - Cited by 38 - Related articles
AIMS Child murder misdiagnosed as sudden infant death syndrome (SIDS) is a ... of areas are
contributing to the decrease in the number of deaths of infants from ... associated with 81
children identified as having been killed by their parents.

Baby Docs: Possible Murder in SIDS Cases - ABC News
https://abcnews.go.com › Health › story ▾
Jan 6, 2006 - While cases of parents killing their babies are rare, more thorough investigations
would probably reveal that some suspected SIDS cases are ...

How Many Babies Really Die of SIDS? - The Atlantic
https://www.theatlantic.com › archive › 2016/06 › understanding-sids ▾
Jun 2, 2016 - Figuring out how many SIDS cases are misclassified may be the key to preventing
it. ... For many parents, the specter of sudden infant death is one of the ... Infant Death
Syndrome, or SIDS, so terrifying, is that it kills newborns ...

Sudden Infant Death Syndrome (SIDS) Symptoms & Causes ...
www.childrenshospital.org › conditions-and-treatments › conditions › sym... ▾
If you're concerned that your child or grandchild is in danger of SIDS, it will comfort you ... of
experience counseling parents on techniques to greatly reduce the risk. ... Diseases caused by
smoking kill almost a half-million people in the United ...

Did these parents accidentally suffocate their children? Or did ...

FIGURE 11.2 (continued)

Typical Parental Responses

Parents tend to struggle most with the answers to three questions after an infant's death [9]. The questions are:

1. Why did this happen?
2. How did this happen to my healthy baby, when I tried so hard to be the best parent I could?
3. What does this mean for my family and future children? How should I parent now?

Interactions with parents will be unpredictable and require patience, understanding, and time. Opportunities arise by simply listening to the questions they have and hearing them tell their stories. Below are suggestions about the framing and focus of your responses to the above questions.

Why Did this Happen?

A response to the question of why the death occurred can be addressed on two separate levels: general information and information specific to their child. Most parents, at some point during this process after their baby has died, will hear someone use the term "SIDS". Most have not thought closely about SIDS and have some very basic questions about what the diagnosis represents. It is not helpful to state that SIDS is a term used when nothing is known—this leaves a parent stranded with endless possibilities and uncontrolled self-blame. There is, however, value in explaining the Triple Risk Model, [10] the prevailing etiologic model for SIDS (see Chap. 2). This multifactorial model is careful to distinguish between risk factors, many of them in the infant's sleep environment, and cause. The Triple Risk Model can be explained by saying that there are three related aspects that converge when an infant dies. The first area of risk involves "extrinsic" risk factors, generally in the infant sleep environment. These associated risk factors are ones they have heard about in anticipatory guidance during the child's healthcare (see Chap. 3). Advice to minimize these risks informs the promotion of safe sleep practices, but generally these are not lethal threats for an infant in any simple sense. The lethality is understood to also involve the contributions from other categories of risk. One category involves maturational aspects of homeostatic mechanisms at ages when infants are especially vulnerable to SIDS, i.e., developmental periods when the incidence of SIDS concentrates. The third component of risk, while not explaining away the importance of associated risk factors in the sleep environment, is "intrinsic" vulnerabilities.

Explaining intrinsic vulnerabilities and speaking with parents about how a seemingly healthy infant could die from inapparent biological vulnerabilities is an important focus for this conversation. Intrinsic vulnerabilities were once understood as largely matters of epidemiologic observations with a biologic basis. Prematurity, low birth weight, maternal smoking, race, or sex all have been found to increase the risk of SIDS and are examples of biologically mediated factors [11]. However, research has increasingly shown that, at least in some cases, the etiology of SIDS involves aberrant arousal and auto-resuscitative mechanisms in an infant [12]. These vulnerabilities have in turn been found to involve brainstem serotonin, its precursors and its transporters, in as many as 70% of SIDS infants [13]. Research based upon this observation has demonstrated terminal mechanisms of failed arousal and cardiorespiratory autoresuscitation consistent with SIDS in serotonin-deficient animal models [14–16]. Other additional neuropathology-based observations include the discovery of "epilepsy in situ", changes otherwise described in epilepsy found in the dentate gyrus of over 40% of infants without a seizure history who have died from SIDS [17]. Moreover, it is estimated that cardiac arrhythmia genes are implicated in 4.3% of SIDS [18].

On a patient level, standard practice in medical examiner systems infrequently yields conclusive diagnostic information about the cause of death. A common gap in the evaluation following SIDS is that an in-person explanation to parents rarely occurs, leaving the family to understand a death certificate and autopsy by themselves. One significant role that primary care providers can play is to review the findings of the autopsy and answer any questions the parents may have. Ideally, this would include the input or attendance of the pathologist performing the autopsy. Family histories, taken with close attention to cardiac, metabolic or epilepsy-related diseases, may also be quite informative about more common diagnostic options for an interested family, and can help inform sensible referrals, although in the US health insurance typically does not cover evaluations for the deceased. For families asking whether further investigation can be pursued, referrals are possible to medical centers with programs that investigate SIDS as an undiagnosed disease, using careful phenotyping and genetic discovery [8]. The contribution made by the careful consideration of potential etiologies using the most current diagnostic methods goes beyond whether a diagnosis is made. Information and stratification of the risk for future SIDS is itself a grief intervention and helps bereaved parents consider their family's future.

How Did this Happen?

The response to the question of how this could happen invites an explanation of modifiable risk factors. This must be answered honestly, yet with an awareness of a parent's psychological dynamics following the death of their child [19]. Many clinicians are wary to directly address specific questions the parents may have, concerned that such topics will be distressing for bereaved parents to discuss even when the parents initiate the conversation. As a general rule, such concerns pale in comparison to the emotional pain of the parents' loss and their desire to better understand it. As one parent said, they will be the parents of a dead baby forever. They are entitled to a frank explanation that is not accusatory but based on the assumption that whatever decisions they made for their child were motivated by their intent to do the best thing for their child at the time.

The answer to how this might have happened involves a sensitive discussion about risk factors in the sleep environment. Risk factors are, in fact, statistically derived associations. Care should be taken to distinguish risk factors from cause unless asphyxia is clearly evident. Nonetheless, a frank discussion of the Triple Risk involves a direct discussion of extrinsic risk. We are unable to ignore the fact that a parent was sharing a sleep surface, for example, no matter how difficult that may be to bring up. At the same time, there is value in divesting them of the idea that they committed infanticide. Care should be taken to explain that it is the view that, except in a small minority of cases, SIDS is not suffocation. Parents also worry that their child suffered as they died. So far as can be known, SIDS occurs quietly and without struggle.

One complicated area is when SIDS occurs in an unaccustomed location or position, which increase the risk for SIDS. Infants may die while in the care of other trusted family members or daycare providers with longstanding relationships to the parents. One in five SIDS deaths in the US occurs in child care centers, approximately one-third in the infant's first week of enrollment [20]. When an infant unaccustomed to prone sleep is placed prone, the risk for SIDS increases by nearly 20-fold [21]. In a case series, the majority of non-prone sleepers dying of SIDS had been changed to prone for the first time, more than half of the time by a non-parent [22]. Sofas are recognized as hazardous locations for infants, but discussing this is more complicated when a parent took a fussy infant to a couch so that the other could sleep.

Parents bereaved after an infant death often confront the stigma associated with these deaths and the insinuation that they have been neglectful, or that the death was caused by some reason the parent would not disclose. In comparison with other deaths after which a young parent will receive great sympathy, parents whose infant has died suddenly and unexpectedly are often socially disenfranchised, and bereavement rituals and supports are often limited [23, 24]. Indeed, the private experiences of parents coupled with the limited opportunities to share their thoughts and feelings without fear of judgment illustrate how social constraints impede post-loss adaptation. This constrained environment contributes to the severity of their grief. This situation is a further argument for the therapeutic value of sensitive explanation and may facilitate their capacity to speak more openly.

Parents may internalize a profound sense of failure and disappointment from their loss. Their psychological state frequently includes self-blame, role confusion, anger, and isolation (Fig. 11.3).

Research has found that more than 45% of mothers after a sudden and unexpected infant death have reported levels of self-blame in the 3 years following their infant's death [25] (Fig. 11.4).

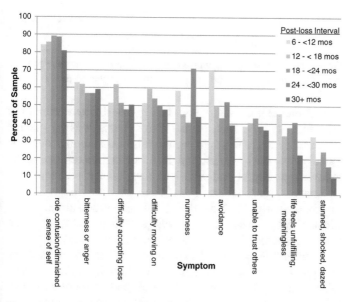

FIGURE 11.3 Cognitive, emotional, and behavioral symptoms of Prolonged Grief Disorder. Symptoms included in diagnostic criteria for PGD shown as percent of time interval sample. Symptoms are highly prevalent and shown in decreasing prevalence. Different patterns of persistence or improvement in specific symptoms can be noted [34].

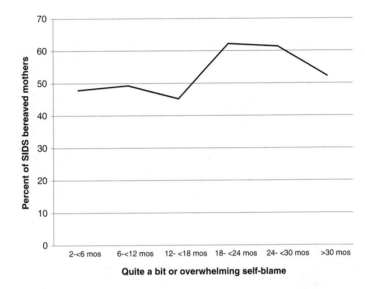

FIGURE 11.4 Self-blame in a cross-sectional study of bereaved mothers 3 years after their infant's sudden and unexpected death

Self-blame is an independent and powerful determinant of grief severity [26]. Parents may blame themselves for specific issues related to the infant's sleep position and environment. Such blame may also extend to other significant areas the parents may regret and wish had been otherwise. Seemingly irrelevant factors will be questioned over and over. Should they have insisted to have their infant examined at the pediatrician's office when they developed congestion and mild URI symptoms? Why did they have such a busy day with their infant? Why were they so motivated to return to work and put their child in daycare? Additionally, some of their self-blame will be rooted in the profound sense of responsibility a parent feels for their child, which unfortunately may never be assuaged by facts or reassurances.

This very difficult environment for loss also contributes to the isolation that is so often reported. Much in the lives of young parents centers on their child and the child's activities. After their infant's death, those same activities and associations may be triggering of grief and distress, and may lead to avoidance. This avoidance extends to peer groups, daily activities, and even social media. Social media, upon which many sudden infant death parent support groups rely to develop communities, can trigger distress and become an object of avoidance. As a group of parents reported, "I don't look at it. Open Facebook and all you see is babies everywhere. All those families looking so happy. And what about those 'one year ago' posts, there to remind us of how much we lost?" Avoidance appears to improve over time, although after 3 years it was reported as a factor in the daily lives of 40% of bereaved mothers (Fig. 11.3).

What Does this Mean Now?

Although parents sometimes change their pediatricians or family physicians after their infant's death, most of the time their relationships with these providers may be the most constant and trusted medical relationships they have during a difficult time. Opportunities to strengthen this relationship arise when their needs are anticipated and you are able to provide some helpful guidance about their future. There is no simple answer to what a parent should take forward after their child's death, nor is there an easy script for anticipatory guidance.

Parents typically want to know whether their infant's death will have any significance for other existing or future children. Reassurance is often provided with the generality: "There is some increased risk for a future infant death but because this is such a rare occurrence in the first place, there is no reason for worry or to let it affect your future family planning, even with that elevated risk." There are two reasons this response fails to meet their needs. The first is the misconception that statistics can genuinely reassure a parent after an unexplained and rare event with such a devastating effect on their lives. For this family, their statistic was 100%. Indeed, perceptions of the estimated likelihood of an unlikely event and its impact are increased in a person after the personal experience of such an event, [27] and evidence demonstrating this can commonly be found in parents after a sudden infant death. Secondly, parents typically look for answers to this question by conducting an independent online search. Those online searches may indicate an elevated risk as much as 10 times greater than in families who have not experienced such a death [28]. It seems better to be in a position to curate their information and contextualize their perceptions of risk.

In a recent study of family risk for unexplained future events after a SIDS death, using U.S. Back to Sleep era data (1995–2013), the risk for SIDS recurrence among siblings was more than quadrupled (odds ratio [OR] 4.2) and increased nearly five-fold for death due to other or unknown causes (OR 4.84). In the extended family, the risk of SIDS recurrence in first- to third-degree relatives of the deceased infant was 9.29 times the risk of the general population [29]. Of course, the actual risk does remain quite small, but the point is that they will find that research documents an increased risk, and that statistical reassurances may have limited effect. This elevated risk also underscores the value of specialized diagnostic programs and the risk stratification they can provide. In this sense, a thorough and exhaustive assessment will either diagnose a disease entity to make the risk better known or will provide additional reassurance because heritable conditions have not been found, thus concretely reducing the odds of a subsequent event.

Parents whose infants die suddenly and unexpectedly may have other living children or may go on to have others. These parents should be given clear messages about the importance of safe sleep. It is hard to imagine a group who will be more receptive to a discussion about sleep environment risks so long as it is offered with sensitivity to the self-blame they likely possess. Beyond sleep advice, parents after an unexpected infant death, as a rule, need more reassurance and help than most others. This is likely to be especially true at the time of birth of any subsequent children, and near the age when their infant died. A more thorough newborn exam, more time with the parents during the birth admission, and a screening electrocardiogram will provide assurances even if they are not especially likely to discover pathology. During routine care, parents may ask many questions seeking reassurances they know are excessive but still find necessary to ask. Providing additional reassurance should not be treated as an indulgence but as a requirement for good care to a family after an infant death. In addition, they will notice when you remember their deceased child during routine healthcare visits for their other children and will especially appreciate it when you use the child's name, as a general rule.

The behavior of parents and their baseline parental anxiety are altered after an infant loss. "Paradoxical parenting" has been described, where parents hover in hypervigilance over the crib of the subsequent infant, while they develop a style of attachment that is more remote or hesitant [30]. This altered attachment is also seen in the fact that a parent with the history of a previous loss will report less severe grief-related symptoms. In caring for subsequent siblings, it can be productive to explain how feeling comfortable and responsive with next newborns after an infant loss can be complicated. They may notice a different feeling from the enchantment they experienced before the loss. Sometimes parents worry about their feelings for the next newborn or feel that positive feelings for the sibling are disloyal to the infant who died. This can become the basis for a discussion about attachment and parenting after losing an infant. It can be helpful to identify the responsibility they may feel to protect the meaning and importance of the deceased infant's life and point out the joy the child would likely have found in siblings.

SIDS (or the other diagnoses frequently used for a sudden unexpected infant death) is a diagnosis made in a setting of acute grief. There are many reasons to anticipate that the severity of the parents' grief will be high. Risk factors for worsened grief include many features seen with these deaths, including a death that (1) is sudden, (2) involves a young infant and (3) involves a relationship with high degrees of dependence on the caregiver [31]. Grief is a psychological reaction rooted in attachment, [32] and the relationship of a parent to their infant is severed at a time of notably high attachment behavior. In most losses, while the symptoms of acute grief may be extreme, information about the death will be processed over time, the finality of the loss will be acknowledged and a new relationship with the deceased will be reconfigured. When this occurs, the bereaved are able to proceed with revised plans, and learn to reinvest in activities and other relationships, regaining a capacity for joy even while a feeling of connectedness with the deceased continues, a connection that includes yearning and emotional pain. This normal grief experience, however, is significantly less common for parents after a sudden and unexpected infant loss.

When severe grief persists beyond 6 months after the infant's death, Prolonged Grief Disorder (PGD) may be present. PGD is diagnosed when grief remains disruptive of daily life beyond 6 months. Its cardinal symptoms are yearning and preoccupation. Other diagnostic elements include role confusion, disbelief, avoidance, intense emotional pain related to the death, difficulty moving on, a feeling the life is meaningless, and intense loneliness (isolation) [33] (Fig. 11.5).

Caution should prevail so as not to pathologize parental grief that, although severe, may be normative. However,

- A significant, disruptive grief response nearly every day for at least the last month
- Characterized by intense **yearning**/longing or **preoccupation** with the deceased person
- And (at least 5):
- **Identity disruption/role confusion**
- **Disbelief** about the death
- **Avoidance** of reminders
- Intense **emotional pain** related to the death
- **Difficulty moving on** with life
- **Emotional numbness**
- Feeling that **life is meaningless**
- Intense **loneliness** (i.e., feeling alone or detached from others

FIGURE 11.5 Current symptomatic criteria for Prolonged Grief Disorder (Proposed DSM-5TR)

given all of the features of the loss noted above, it should be no surprise that nearly 60% of mothers had PGD at 1 year following their infant's death, and over 40% had PGD 3 years after the loss [34]. Indeed, two-thirds of parents report the death of their child as affecting their daily life in important ways 12–15 years later [35]. This is significant in itself, but also because such grief can affect a household and other children. These other children may be in your practice.

Opportunities can arise by investigating cognitive or behavioral aspects of more severe grief. In research on mothers after a sudden and unexpected infant death, the majority of mothers had high and persistent levels of role confusion, diminished sense of self, bitterness or anger. Difficulty moving on and an inability to trust others are also persistent and unresolving (Fig. 11.5). This may be especially true in mothers with a history of depression, alcohol use or in older mothers [36]. Parents with other children in the home often express gratitude that other children pull them out of their grief, although our research suggests that the advantages are short lived [36]. All of these topics are worth exploring and may be helpful to a parent's post-loss adaptation.

Support groups with other parents who have been similarly bereaved have unique benefits, their shared experiences allowing newly bereaved parents to escape the stigma or feel that the particular shock of their loss is recognized. The groups offer a supportive environment to share their stories and experiences, validate their feelings and lessen their sense of isolation. Referrals to these programs can be obtained by contacting national SIDS/SUID parent organizations or organizations dedicated to support parents whose children have died (see Resources section for additional details). Individual therapy sessions can also be of great help, especially if the therapist has experience with parental loss of a very young child. Encouraging parents to develop and maintain routines is a sound recommendation to offer. Loss can cause a physical quarantine in addition to psychological isolation, and the loss of regular activities is known to worsen grief [37]. There is also a physical component to grief that may surprise a parent with its persistence, manifesting as exercise intolerance or fatigue. It is helpful to remind parents to practice self-care, especially those who must return quickly to work and face emotional exhaustion. Another helpful area to explore is friendships and trusted supports, which frequently change during this time of great need because of disappointing responses. It is easy for parents to focus on the loss and disappointment, but they should also be encouraged to assemble a protective group who have been present and who can be relied upon. Somewhat relatedly, taking an active role in assuring for legacies and remembrances gives occasion for others to remember their child and hear people speaking the child's name, while providing new opportunities for creating support systems. Such legacy building should be encouraged.

For many bereaved parents, the extended family is a tremendous resource and offers safety and a willingness to provide concrete help that is usually supportive and practical. Yet, relationships with the extended family can be stressed by a parent's experiences during an infant loss. Members of the extended family sometimes need to be reminded that there is no set time for a bereaved parent to "get over" the loss. Rather, the task is to learn to tolerate and accommodate its presence in their lives. While denial or avoidance of anything to do with the deceased child is not helpful, it should also be recognized that many family events present difficult challenges and can feel very alienating to the recently bereaved. There may be a time in their bereavement when celebrating or diversion feels impossible or like a betrayal to their deceased infant. They may find themselves "faking it" through events while feeling despair within. Spending time with other small children, including nieces and nephews who were born when their deceased child was born or are at ages that remind them of their deceased child, can be complicated. It is helpful for parents to develop a plan for how much time to spend in these situations and have an "exit strategy."

It can be useful to explain that parents in couples grieve differently and interdependently. Avoidance of discussion about their experiences of loss and trying to appear strong to protect their partner is associated with higher levels of grief in both [38]. Moreover, there is more grief when a parent does not trust that their partner will be emotionally present and available at a time of need [39]. The struggle is for each member of a couple to grieve in a way that is authentic while also supporting and helping one another through an uncertain and overwhelming time. Setting time aside on a regular basis to check in with each other about their grieving experiences creates a space to speak more freely without worrying that they will upset the other.

Despite all of the challenges a young family confronts after an infant loss, it is important to keep sight of the strength and personal motivation that parents manage to summon. At extraordinary cost, they have learned deep lessons about the fragility and preciousness of life. They have confronted the profound obligations of parenthood and the meaning of a life. For those who pause to notice it, those who have been helped in the aftermath of their loss and who have somehow managed through it will bring unique strengths to their family in the future. The loss will never go away, but efforts to honor the child can leave a beautiful mark.

In conclusion, coping after the terrible loss from the sudden and unexpected death of an infant is an isolating and extremely difficult experience for parents. Most of their relationships are tested during this time, including their relationships with their pediatricians or family physicians. Concrete contributions from the health care provider include guiding the family through the system and advocating for their need to find answers. Because of the privileged access a provider has with a young family, and the few other medical supports typically in their lives, counseling about grief and helping them anticipate solutions to social complexities will help the family. In any interaction, assessing their coping, saying their child's name, and letting them tell their story will have therapeutic value.

Vignette Follow-Up

Several weeks after Zach's death, their pediatrician invited Bill and Ayanna into the office to see how they were coping and to understand ways she could be helpful. She scheduled the meeting after office hours to reduce the triggers that might remind them of their loss. At the appointment, they appreciated her concern but also her non-judgmental explanation about what is known and not known about SUID. She asked them what they were most worried about that might be related to Zach's death. She listened and was careful in how she offered reassurances. They could see that their pediatrician was disturbed by Zach's death and found that comforting somehow. They were glad she did not burden them by allowing that distress to become a focus but instead kept the focus on them.

Although she didn't have all the answers, they appreciated being able to talk with someone who knew them as a family before Zach's death. They felt less defensive and were more able to honestly express their complicated feelings and concerns. They were relieved when she offered to communicate with the medical examiner on their behalf and to help them understand the death certificate when it was completed. They were grateful that she recognized what a profound, lasting challenge Zach's death posed for them as individuals, parents, and as a family, and her earnest desire to help find ways for them to seek more answers and be supported in their grief.

Clinical Pearls

- Parents are wounded by their loss, and that has implications for the entire household, including other children.
- The physician role is not to stand in judgment but to help them accommodate to their loss.
- Mediating with the system is protective and helpful.
- There are answers that can be provided to help make the event more understandable.

- Advocating for higher levels of diagnostic efforts sometimes yields results and always has a positive effect on grief.
- Pursue questions that parents may have about what the death means for their other children.
- There are ways to make grief more knowable and less overwhelming to parents.

References

1. Garstang J, Griffiths F, Sidebotham P. What do bereaved parents want from professionals after the sudden death of their child: a systematic review of the literature. BMC Pediatr. 2014;14:269. PMCID: PMC4287432. Epub 2014/10/15.
2. Camperlengo L, Shapiro-Mendoza CK, Gibbs F. Improving sudden unexplained infant death investigation practices: an evaluation of the Centers for Disease Control and Prevention's SUID Investigation Training Academies. Am J Forensic Med Pathol. 2014;35(4):278–82.
3. Fleming PJ, Blair PS, Sidebotham PD, Hayler T. Investigating sudden unexpected deaths in infancy and childhood and caring for bereaved families: an integrated multiagency approach. BMJ. 2004;328(7435):331–4. PMCID: PMC338105.
4. Mitchell RA, DiAngelo C, Morgan D. Medicolegal Death Investigation of sudden unexpected infant deaths. Pediatr Ann. 2017;46(8):e297–e302.
5. Erck Lambert AB, Parks SE, Camperlengo L, Cottengim C, Anderson RL, Covington TM, et al. Death Scene Investigation and autopsy practices in sudden unexpected infant deaths. J Pediatr. 2016;174:84–90.e1. PMCID: PMC5063238. Epub 2016/04/22.
6. Petrikin JE, Willig LK, Smith LD, Kingsmore SF. Rapid whole genome sequencing and precision neonatology. Seminars in perinatology. 2015;39(8):623–31. PMCID: PMC4657860. Epub 2015/11/02.
7. The National Association of Medical Examiners. NAME Inspection and Accreditation Checklist. 2018. p. 23.
8. Goldstein RD, Nields HM, Kinney HC. A New approach to the investigation of sudden unexpected death. Pediatrics. 2017;140(2):e20170024.

9. Martin K. When a baby dies of SIDS: the parents' grief and search for reason. New York: Routledge; 2016.

10. Filiano JJ, Kinney HC. A perspective on neuropathologic findings in victims of the sudden infant death syndrome: the triple-risk model. Biol Neonate. 1994;65(3–4):194–7.

11. Moon RY, Task Force On Sudden Infant Death S. SIDS and other sleep-related infant deaths: evidence base for 2016 updated recommendations for a safe infant sleeping environment. Pediatrics. 2016;138(5):e20162940.

12. Kinney HC, Thach BT. The sudden infant death syndrome. N Engl J Med. 2009;361(8):795–805. PMCID: 3268262.

13. Kinney HC, Richerson GB, Dymecki SM, Darnall RA, Nattie EE. The brainstem and serotonin in the sudden infant death syndrome. Ann Rev Pathol. 2009;4:517–50. PMCID: 3268259.

14. Cummings KJ, Commons KG, Hewitt JC, Daubenspeck JA, Li A, Kinney HC, et al. Failed heart rate recovery at a critical age in 5-HT-deficient mice exposed to episodic anoxia: implications for SIDS. J Appl Physiol. 2011;111(3):825–33. PMCID: 3174796.

15. Cummings KJ, Hewitt JC, Li A, Daubenspeck JA, Nattie EE. Postnatal loss of brainstem serotonin neurones compromises the ability of neonatal rats to survive episodic severe hypoxia. J Physiol. 2011;589(Pt 21):5247–56. PMCID: 3225677.

16. Dosumu-Johnson RT, Cocoran AE, Chang Y, Nattie E, Dymecki SM. Acute perturbation of Pet1-neuron activity in neonatal mice impairs cardiorespiratory homeostatic recovery. eLife. 2018;7. PMCID: PMC6199134. Epub 2018/10/24.

17. Kinney HC, Cryan JB, Haynes RL, Paterson DS, Haas EA, Mena OJ, et al. Dentate gyrus abnormalities in sudden unexplained death in infants: morphological marker of underlying brain vulnerability. Acta Neuropathol. 2015;129(1):65–80. PMCID: 4282685.

18. Tester DJ, Wong LCH, Chanana P, Jaye A, Evans JM, FitzPatrick DR, et al. Cardiac genetic predisposition in sudden infant death syndrome. J Am Coll Cardiol. 2018;71(11):1217–27.

19. Morris S, Fletcher K, Goldstein R. The grief of parents after the death of a young child. J Clin Psychol Med Settings. 2018;26(3):321–38. Epub 2018/11/30

20. Moon RY, Patel KM, Shaefer SJ. Sudden infant death syndrome in child care settings. Pediatrics. 2000;106(2 Pt 1):295–300.

21. Mitchell EA, Thach BT, Thompson JM, Williams S. Changing infants' sleep position increases risk of sudden infant death

syndrome. New Zealand Cot Death Study. Arch Pediatr Adolesc Med. 1999;153(11):1136–41. Epub 1999/11/11

22. Cote A, Gerez T, Brouillette RT, Laplante S. Circumstances leading to a change to prone sleeping in sudden infant death syndrome victims. Pediatrics. 2000;106(6):E86. Epub 2000/01/11

23. Juth V, Smyth JM, Carey MP, Lepore SJ. Social constraints are associated with negative psychological and physical adjustment in bereavement. Appl Psychol Health Well Being. 2015;7(2):129–48. Epub 2015/02/24

24. Lepore SJ, Silver RC, Wortman CB, Wayment HA. Social constraints, intrusive thoughts, and depressive symptoms among bereaved mothers. J Pers Soc Psychol. 1996;70(2):271–82.

25. Goldstein RD. Unpublished data from NIH ancillary study, Maternal Grief in High Risk Settings. 2016.

26. Stroebe M, Stroebe W, van de Schoot R, Schut H, Abakoumkin G, Li J. Guilt in bereavement: the role of self-blame and regret in coping with loss. PloS One. 2014;9(5):e96606. PMCID: PMC4018291. Epub 2014/05/14.

27. Erev I, Glozman I, Hertwig R. What impacts the impact of rare events. J Risk Uncertain. 2008;36(2):153–77.

28. Hunt CE. Sudden infant death syndrome and other causes of infant mortality: diagnosis, mechanisms, and risk for recurrence in siblings. Am J Respir Crit Care Med. 2001;164(3):346–57.

29. Christensen ED, Berger J, Alashari MM, Coon H, Robison C, Ho HT, et al. Sudden infant death "syndrome"-insights and future directions from a Utah population database analysis. Am J Med Genet A. 2017;173(1):177–82. Epub 2016/10/30

30. Warland J, O'Leary J, McCutcheon H, Williamson V. Parenting paradox: parenting after infant loss. Midwifery. 2011;27(5):e163–9.

31. Morris S, Fletcher K, Goldstein R. The grief of parents after the death of a young child. J Clin Psychol Med Settings. 2019;26(3):321–38. Epub 2018/11/30

32. Bowlby J. Attachment and loss: retrospect and prospect. Am J Orthopsychiatry. 1982;52(4):664–78. Epub 1982/10/01

33. Prigerson HG, Horowitz MJ, Jacobs SC, Parkes CM, Aslan M, Goodkin K, et al. Prolonged grief disorder: psychometric validation of criteria proposed for DSM-V and ICD-11. PLoS Med. 2009;6(8):e1000121. PMCID: PMC2711304.

34. Goldstein RD, Lederman RI, Lichtenthal WG, Morris SE, Human M, Elliott AJ, et al. The grief of mothers after the sudden unexpected death of their infants. Pediatrics. 2018;141(5):e20173651.

35. Dyregrov A, Dyregrov K. Long-term impact of sudden infant death: a 12- to 15-year follow-up. Death Stud. 1999;23(7):635–61.
36. Goldstein RD, Petty CR, Morris SE, Human M, Odendaal H, Elliott A, et al. Pre-loss personal factors and prolonged grief disorder in bereaved mothers. Psychol Med. 2018;9:1–9. Epub 2018/11/10
37. Hofer MA. Relationships as regulators: a psychobiologic perspective on bereavement. Psychosom Med. 1984;46(3):183–97.
38. Stroebe M, Finkenauer C, Wijngaards-de Meij L, Schut H, van den Bout J, Stroebe W. Partner-oriented self-regulation among bereaved parents: the costs of holding in grief for the partner's sake. Psychol Sci. 2013;24(4):395–402.
39. Wijngaards-de Meij L, Stroebe M, Schut H, Stroebe W, van den Bout J, van der Heijden PG, et al. Parents grieving the loss of their child: interdependence in coping. Br J Clin Psychol. 2008;47(Pt 1):31–42.

Chapter 12
Advocating for Safe Sleep

Samuel Hanke and Rachel Y. Moon

The impact of the American Academy of Pediatrics "Back to Sleep" recommendations in the mid-1990s was dramatic and undeniable. The simple message to place babies on their back for sleep resulted in behavior change in millions of families, and this behavior change was associated with a dramatic decline in sleep-related infant deaths over the next decade. Unfortunately, the behavior changes and decreased mortality experienced with the Back to Sleep campaign have not been replicated in the [1–5] "Safe to Sleep" recommendations released in 2011. Since the initial decline in mortality rates, rates have remained stubbornly stagnant. Indeed, there have been recent increases in non-supine positioning and bedsharing, use of soft bedding remains at >50%, and breastfeeding rates at 6 months remain low.

The factors that influence these stagnant rates are numerous, complex, and the subject of intense academic inquiry. As health care providers, we now must navigate multiple sources of information, misinformation, and societal factors that

S. Hanke (✉)
Heart Institute, Cincinnati Children's Hospital Medical Center, Cincinnati, OH, USA
e-mail: Samuel.hanke@cchmc.org

R. Y. Moon
Department of Pediatrics, University of Virginia School of Medicine, Charlottesville, VA, USA

© Springer Nature Switzerland AG 2020
R. Y. Moon (ed.), *Infant Safe Sleep*,
https://doi.org/10.1007/978-3-030-47542-0_12

influence infant sleep choice. Many of these factors are not rooted in sound scientific inquiry and understanding of risk. Effectively advocating for our infants requires an understanding of this complex interplay.

Emotion Trumps Reason

The big question is: Why are parents choosing to take on risk by placing their baby in a more dangerous environment? While we have become skilled at messaging the "what's" of safe sleep, we still have not clearly communicated the "why" or "how." Are parents choosing to take on this additional risk because the statistics aren't "real" enough and the risk is theoretical? Is the risk too general and not personalized enough? Is parents' risk "literacy" too low? Risk literacy is one's practical ability to evaluate and understand risk, and to use this understanding when making decisions. Interestingly, risk literacy strongly correlates with practical understanding of mathematics. For instance, many people are much more scared to get into an airplane than a car, because they are worried about a plane crash. In reality, you are more likely to die in a car on your way to the airport than you are to die in the plane. In 2017, 399 people died in plane crashes worldwide, compared with >37,000 who died in car crashes in the United States alone [6]. This is an example of low-risk literacy. Part of this is because people generally think that the frequency of an occurrence is related to how quickly one can think of that occurrence [7]. One can easily recall at least as many plane crashes as car crashes. After all, plane crashes are always covered in the news, and because one is always hearing about them, one assumes that they occur frequently.

Equally or more important than risk literacy is the psychology of risk. Famous NYU Neuroscientist and brain researcher Joseph Ledoux published extensively about the emotional brain and how our brain processes fear and emotion [8]. Two important conclusions from his work are that (1) our brain is hard-wired to feel first and think second, and (2) emotion and instinct readily and easily overwhelm conscious and purposeful reasoning. The immediate distress that a parent feels when the baby keeps crying may be more important at the moment than an abstract risk of the infant dying suddenly and unexpectedly, and the parent may place the baby on the stomach.

Our parents are facing numerous factors influencing their choice and behavior. Many of these, including the influences of social norms, baby comfort, maternal comfort, crib availability, fatigue, convenience, advice, and modeling from health care professionals, and then finally their understanding of the risk associated with their choice, have already been discussed in this book.

Advocacy to Health Care Providers

To Influence Others, We Must First Influence Ourselves

Parents trust medical providers. A 2018 Gallup poll asked over 1000 Americans what professions are the most trusted in terms of honesty and ethical standards. The top three professions (nurses, medical doctors, pharmacists) are the core of the public-facing medical community. Yet when surveyed in 2012, only 43% of pediatricians and 38% of the pediatric residents report "never co-sleeping" with their own infants [9]. How as a medical community can we expect effective advocacy if we are unable to practice what we preach?

Eisenberg and colleagues surveyed mothers of infants age 2–6 months of age regarding the advice they received from physicians, birth hospital nurses, family and media regarding sleep position, sleep location, and pacifier use. Over 50% reported no advice from physicians regarding sleep location and pacifier use, and 20% received no advice for sleep position. Even more alarming, an additional 25% received advice that was not consistent with the AAP safe sleep recommendations [10].

To effectively advocate for safe sleep, we must first advocate for safe sleep within the health care community—among the doctors, nurses, and allied health staff who have their own children. Comprehensive safe sleep training should be required curriculum in medical and nursing schools. It should be further reinforced in pediatric, family medicine, and obstetrics-gynecology residency programs.

This education should not only address the evidence-based recommendations from the AAP but also discuss conflicting infant sleep recommendations from other health care societies. While the majority of the recommendations are consistent (i.e., back to sleep, tobacco and alcohol avoidance, and no infant sleep on sofas, armchairs, or pillows) there are important differences in the interpreted risks and benefits of bedsharing [11]. Most notably, there has been controversy about whether the benefits of bedsharing (facilitating breastfeeding) outweigh the risks of SUID while bedsharing (see Chap. 6 for a detailed discussion). When recommendations are inconsistent, parents are more confused and less likely to follow safe sleep practices.

Advocacy Within the Community

Despite data supporting the importance of a consistent health care message from all sectors of society in changing practice norms, it is increasingly difficult to sustain a consistent health care message. A recent example of success in this regard is the change in cigarette smoking. Thirty years ago, smoking was considered acceptable and even normal in some US communities. However, with concerted efforts from the health care community, lawmakers, and others, laws were passed to prohibit smoking in public areas, children were educated in health classes about the dangers of smoking, and cigarette advertisements disappeared and were replaced by public service announcements about the consequences of smoking. The social norm changed such that smoking rates decreased from 42.6% in 1965 to 14% in

2017, and there is more of a social stigma if one is a cigarette smoker [12].

Unfortunately, our modern society has made such a unified health care message much more difficult. The internet makes misinformation readily available. We can see this on a daily basis with regards to vaccines. Despite consistent messaging within the health care community and strong supporting evidence for vaccination, alternative, vocal, and widely disseminated anti-vaccination messages have increased rates of vaccine hesitancy and anti-vaccine sentiment and negatively impacted immunization rates, resulting in recurrence of vaccine-preventable diseases. Part of the wide acceptance of anti-vaccination messages comes from the overwhelming success of vaccines. When one does not believe that one's child is at risk for getting a deadly vaccine-preventable disease, one is less likely to believe that a vaccine is necessary. Safe sleep has also been a victim of success. When parents hear that SIDS rates have declined—and when they do not hear much about SIDS in the news—they assume that this is a problem that has gone away and thus a threat that they do not need to worry about. When we advocate for infant safe sleep, we have to remember the lessons learned from past public health campaigns and consider the influences that are important in parental decision-making (See Chap. 4).

Behavior change requires a change in social norms. If there are constant images of babies sleeping prone or cribs stuffed with bedding, these create a perception that "everyone is doing it"—i.e., a social norm. We can start changing these perceived norms by assuring that marketing materials are consistent with safe sleep guidelines. Look at advertisements in your Sunday newspaper. One study found that only half of magazine advertisements for infant cribs and sleep products portrayed a safe sleep environment [13]. You can even just start with advertisements in medical journals; it is surprising how many medical institutions use images of babies in unsafe sleep environments in their advertising. This is partly due to the fact that most advertisements will use stock photographs for their images; one study that looked at 1590 stock photographs of sleeping infants found that <40% of the infants were portrayed in the supine position, and only 5% of the photographs depicted a safe sleep environment [14]! *When you see unsafe sleep environments depicted, you can contact the company directly or contact the publication to alert them.* Let them know that the 4A's (aaaa.org), a national organization of advertising and marketing agencies, has advertising guidelines for safe sleep images [15].

Similarly, when you see products that are not aligned with safe sleep recommendations, these also create a perception that these products are acceptable to use. Most parents do not realize that there are no safety standards for most of these products, and that there is no regulatory agency that vets these products before they are sold. Parents assume that if baby products are being sold, they must be safe. Contact the manufacturers of these products to let them know that they are unsafe. Speak out on the company's social media platforms, so that others can see that there are safety concerns with the product.

We also need to use these platforms and a marketing mindset to communicate best safe sleep practices and tips. How can we use creative and effective marketing strategies to not only communicate but change behaviors when it comes to safe sleep? Connecting with marketing professionals to develop attractive, shareable messaging is a great place to start.

Recognize that the insatiable consumption of content in the 24-hour-news-cycle-world in which we are living means that consumers are able to track down content that fits their belief systems. Thus, we need to use these platforms to share evidence-based information. In this digital age, it is perhaps even more important to assure that the content is not only scientifically correct, but broadly appealing and highly shareable. The more a message is reposted, shared and liked, the more engagement it generates; these good stories can go "viral."

We can use marketing in the same way large companies use it to sell their products. Think about a message that uses humor and empathy, or tugs on heartstrings. Understand what it is you are trying to accomplish with each message or campaign. Am I trying to inform? Promote an idea? What are my values when it comes to my practice or organization? How can I communicate these values when it comes to safe sleep?

In addition to social media, consider other tools you can use to share safe sleep messages to back up your online efforts. These marketing strategies can include billboards, sides of buses, ads on the radio, television or streaming platforms. Safe sleep content can also be shared using editorial appeals rather than advertising. Consider an article or blog post, as that may be more effective or "believable" to the consumer than an ad on that same site.

Remember that there is power in numbers. Find organizations and individuals with whom you can partner. In several communities, first responders are trained to provide safe sleep education to families; when they respond to a 911 call (even if it is for an adult with chest pain), they assess the home for an infant and the infant's sleep environment, and they provide safe sleep information on the spot [16]. Parents who have lost an infant are powerful forces, as they represent a subset which can contextualize the risk associated with on safe sleep and provide their stories to support the message. Connect with faith leaders, sports and entertainment figures, and other respected community leaders to send a consistent message and create a community norm of safe sleep.

Advocating for Policy Change

Laws that ensure car seat safety have existed for years. We won't let a baby leave the hospital until we see that she is being properly secured in a car seat. At every doctor's visit from that point on, parents are asked about car seats—and that vigilance is saving lives. With increased knowledge to the public, better surveillance, and innovative safety technologies, the number of child deaths in motor vehicle crashes has dropped by over half in the last 20 years [17].

This widespread adoption of car safety standards is easy to understand when you take a look at your own commitment to car safety. Chances are high that you rode in a car today. Additionally, chances are that, while going from home to work or to the dry cleaner, you didn't get in a car wreck. Without thinking about it, you habitually buckled yourself and your children, because the chances of death via motor vehicle crash are a lot less likely when you are wearing a seat belt (adult) or in the appropriately sized car seat (child). The seat belt or car seat doesn't guarantee survival if something catastrophic happens, but it significantly increases your chances for a safe arrival. (Of course, in addition to safety concerns there is the added motivator of legal consequences should you get caught without proper restraints for you and your children.)

Lower death rates as a result of seat belt safety laws prove that the widespread adoption of car safety practices is working. In 2017, 91 infants died in car crashes in the United States. In that same year, 3641 infants died of sudden unexpected infant death [17]. While there are no laws that allow us access into a family's home we can share this analogy. When talking with new parents, ask them commit to absolute standards of safety for safe sleep, just as they commit to absolute standards of automotive safety. Safe sleep gives infants the greatest chance to wake up.

The challenge is that we can't regulate what goes on behind closed doors. So, how can we influence behavior with policy change for an activity that takes place almost wholly within the walls of someone's home? We can start by eliminating products with known safety concerns. In the fall of 2019 the Consumer Product Safety Commission called for a halt in sales of all inclined sleepers. Over the next several months, they issued recalls trying to eliminate these products from the marketplace and people's homes. Sadly, many of the products are still available secondhand or passed down from older children. It is important for medical professionals to be aware of such product dangers and share the information with parents.

While the CPSC is an important agency in assessing the safety of products, lawmakers still need to get involved in these issues to help enforce standards. In December 2019, the U.S. House of Representatives passed the Safe Sleep for Babies Act of 2019 (H.R. 3172). This legislation, if passed by the Senate and signed into law, would ban infant inclined sleep products and padded crib bumper pads.

In addition to laws regarding product safety, a standard of care needs to be formally established for the investigation and classifications of infant deaths. Laws requiring better death scene data would lead to a better understanding of SUID deaths and would therefore lead to better education. Such a law was introduced by Senator Bob Casey in 2019. Known as the Scarlett's Sunshine Act, the law would strengthen existing efforts to better understand sudden unexpected deaths in infants and children, facilitate data collection and analysis to improve prevention efforts, and support children and families.

While we wait for lawmakers to help us in our efforts to establish absolute standards of safety and reporting, we must be the "boots on the ground" messengers of such valuable information. We have a duty to our patients to discuss the limitations of lawmakers and regulatory agencies when it comes to product safety and infant care. We can be the voice and the advocates for the infants in our charge. Speaking up and understanding what is happening in our patients' homes is a great first step. Staying up to date on the latest product recalls and legislation as it relates to safe sleep can lead to better communication with and information for our families, and ultimately better outcomes.

It Is All Our Responsibility

We all have a role to play in helping new parents be successful by recognizing the challenges that come with practicing safe sleep starting with nurses modeling safe sleep in the delivery hospital, to the pediatrician offering real practical tips on getting newborns to sleep, to the friend that can hold the baby so mom and dad can get a break, to the firefighter recognizing an unsafe sleep environment when on an ambulance run, to the child care provider making sure every crib in their facility is blanket and pillow free.

Providing solutions and support can empower parents to follow through with their safe sleep plan. So parents, don't be afraid to ask for help. Friends, be encouraging and tell new parents they are doing a great job. Grandparents, be supportive and lend a hand when possible. And finally, all of us can lead with empathy and share real stories from those that have been impacted by sleep-related deaths.

References

1. Colson ER, Willinger M, Rybin D, Heeren T, Smith LA, Lister G, et al. Trends and factors associated with infant bed sharing, 1993–2010: the National Infant Sleep Position Study. JAMA Pediatr. 2013;167(11):1032–7.
2. Colson ER, Rybin D, Smith LA, Colton T, Lister G, Corwin MJ. Trends and factors associated with infant sleeping position: the national infant sleep position study, 1993–2007. Arch Pediatr Adolesc Med. 2009;163(12):1122–8.
3. Shapiro-Mendoza CK, Colson ER, Willinger M, Rybin DV, Camperlengo L, Corwin MJ. Trends in infant bedding use: National Infant Sleep Position study, 1993–2010. Pediatrics. 2015;135(1):10–7.
4. Centers for Disease Control and Prevention, National Immunization Surveys.
5. Hirai AH, Kortsmit K, Kaplan L, Reiney E, Warner L, Parks SE, Shapiro-Mendoza CK. Prevalence and factors associated with safe infant sleep practices. Pediatrics. 2019;144(5).

6. Bureau of Aircraft Accidents Archives. Available from: https://web.archive.org/web/20170712212958/http://www.baaa-acro.com/general-statistics/death-rate-per-year/.

7. Kahneman D. Thinking, fast and slow (1st pbk. ed.). New York: Farrar, Straus and Giroux; New York, NY. 2013.

8. LeDoux J. The emotional brain: the mysterious underpinnings of emotional life. Simon and Schuster; 1998.

9. Wheeler J, O'Riordan M, Solomon J. Do pediatric residents and attending physicians practice what they preach? Clin Pediatr. 2013;52(12):1176–7.

10. Eisenberg SR, Bair-Merritt MH, Colson ER, Heeren TC, Geller NL, Corwin MJ. Maternal report of advice received for infant care. Pediatrics. 2015;136(2):e315–e22.

11. Blair PS, Ball HL, McKenna JJ, Feldman-Winter L, Marinelli KA, Bartick MC, et al. Bedsharing and breastfeeding: the academy of breastfeeding medicine protocol# 6, revision 2019. Breastfeeding Med. 2020.

12. American Lung Association. Available from: https://www.lung.org/our-initiatives/research/monitoring-trends-in-lung-disease/tobacco-trend-brief/overall-tobacco-trends.html.

13. Kreth M, Shikany T, Lenker C, Troxler RB. Safe sleep guideline adherence in nationwide marketing of infant cribs and products. Pediatrics. 2017;139(1):e20161729.

14. Goodstein MH, Lagon E, Bell T, Joyner BL, Moon RY. Stock photographs do not comply with infant safe sleep guidelines. Clin Pediatr. 2018;57(4):403–9.

15. 4A's Guidance Paper: Safe-Sleep Image Advertising Guidelines. Available from: https://www.aaaa.org/index.php?checkfileaccess=/wp-content/uploads/legacy-pdfs/SafeSleep11-17-14_FINAL.pdf.

16. Moon RY, Hauck FR, Colson ER. Safe infant sleep interventions: what is the evidence for successful behavior change? Curr Pediatr Rev. 2016;12(1):67–75.

17. Centers for Disease Control and Prevention. Available from: https://wonder.cdc.gov/ucd-icd10.html.

Helpful Resources

Please note that this list of resources is not comprehensive. There are other websites that have helpful information for providers and families. Additionally, it should be noted that these websites are geared toward the US audience. There are often similar resources in other countries.

SIDS/SUID Educational Resources:

- American Academy of Pediatrics:

  - The AAP's safe sleep webpage has links to policy statements and recent publications regarding safe sleep guidelines. It also has links to purchase parent education brochures. https://www.aap.org/en-us/advocacy-and-policy/aap-health-initiatives/child_death_review/Pages/Safe-Sleep.aspx.

  - The AAP's breastfeeding webpage has links to policy statements and recent publications regarding breastfeeding. https://www.aap.org/en-us/advocacy-and-policy/aap-health-initiatives/Breastfeeding/Pages/default.aspx.

  - The AAP also sponsors a parenting website that has additional resources: www.healthychildren.org.

- American SIDS Institute: The American SIDS Institute provides educational materials, bereavement support, and research support. https://sids.org/

- Centers for Disease Control and Prevention: The CDC's sudden unexpected infant death and sudden infant death

© Springer Nature Switzerland AG 2020
R. Y. Moon (ed.), *Infant Safe Sleep*,
https://doi.org/10.1007/978-3-030-47542-0

syndrome webpage provides information about SUID and SIDS, data, and statistics. There are also educational resources for parents and information about infant death investigations. https://www.cdc.gov/sids/index.htm

- Safe to Sleep campaign: The Safe to Sleep campaign is sponsored by the National Institutes of Health. This webpage has many helpful education resources. https://safetosleep.nichd.nih.gov/
- Cribs for Kids: Cribs for Kids is an organization that partners with programs across the USA to provide low-cost or free portable cribs to families who otherwise would not be able to afford a safe sleep space for their infant. https://cribsforkids.org/
- National Center for Education in Maternal and Child Health at Georgetown University has developed a "Conversations Approach" to gain knowledge and skills needed to answer parent questions in support of both breastfeeding and safe sleep practices. https://www.ncemch.org/learning/building/

Bereavement Support Resources:

- First Candle is a national organization that provides bereavement support for families who have experienced an infant loss. They have information about parent support groups and educational materials for families. https://firstcandle.org/
- The Compassionate Friends is a national organization that provides bereavement support to families who have experienced infant or child loss. https://www.compassionatefriends.org/

Product Safety Resources:

- The US Consumer Product Safety Commission provides information about product safety standards that are in effect. (Note: there are many products for which there are no standards.) Recall information can be found at https://

cpsc.gov/Recalls. In addition, complaints or concerns about any product, whether there has been a true incident/accident or there is concern about a potential incident/accident, can be reported at https://www.saferproducts.gov/CPSRMSPublic/Incidents/ReportIncident.aspx.

Index

© Springer Nature Switzerland AG 2020   261
R. Y. Moon (ed.), *Infant Safe Sleep*,
https://doi.org/10.1007/978-3-030-47542-0

Printed in the United States
By Bookmasters